Letters From The Land of Long Farewells

Kalaupapa, Molokai

Sister Wilma Halmasy, O.S.F.

DEDICATED TO THE SISTERS OF ST. FRANCIS WHO HAVE SERVED AT KALAUPAPA

"We carried the touch of Hope in the early days and we didn't hope in vain."

These poignant words written by Sister Wilma Halmasy convey well the spirit of the dedicated Franciscan Sisters of Syracuse, New York, who brought their ministry of loving nursing care, good management and proper housing to the exiled residents of Kalaupapa beginning in the year 1888. The example of the strong faith of the Sisters in a merciful God and their presence in otherwise dismal surroundings brought hope and comfort to those confined to the settlement. The longtime hoped-for blessing of a means of healing allowing the residents to be free from confinement came about eventually with the coming to the settlement of new drugs in 1946.

SISTER WILMA HALMASY AND THE FRANCISCAN SISTERS' CONTINUATION OF THE LEGACY OF MOTHER MARIANNE COPE

Sixty-one Sisters of St. Francis of Syracuse have worked for the Department of Health in Hawaii at Kalaupapa, Molokai, caring for those afflicted with leprosy, now called Hansen's Disease. The work of the Sisters began with their beloved and heroically virtuous leader, Mother Marianne Cope, in November 1888.

Sister Wilma Halmasy, the author of this charming and insightful book of letters, lived at the settlement for thirty years. Sister served devotedly as a nurse in the mid 1940s, and in later decades, as the supervisor of the Department of Health at the Kalaupapa Hospital. Her descriptions reveal the daily life of the sisters and residents at Kalaupapa during her time. Like others who have been privileged to read her letters, the reader will delight in Sister's handling of distressful and sometimes amusing situations. Sister Wilma's courage as well as the courage of those serving with her at the isolated Kalaupapa peninsula will be startling and inspirational to the reader.

Sister Wilma in giving testimony in the 1980s for Mother Marianne's Cause of Canonization wrote: "Mother continued to think of her charges to the end; her motto was do all for the love of God." This work of art by Sister Wilma displays in a heartfelt manner the deep love the sisters from Mother Marianne down to the present sisters continue to have for the people of Kalaupapa today.

This is a true story worth reading.

A BIOGRAPHICAL NOTE

Sister Wilma was well enough to attend Mother Marianne's beatification in May 2005. Sister was called to her eternal reward a year afterward on June 24, 2006. She died at the age of 85 in Syracuse, New York.

Sister Wilma was born Lillian Halmasy to Julius and Mary Baumgartner Halmasy, both Hungarian immigrants, in Lorain, Ohio, on February 9, 1921.

She entered the community of the Sisters of St. Francis on September 8, 1937 from her home parish of St. Mary in Akron, Ohio. She was invested as a Franciscan Sister in 1938 and made her final vows in 1943. Sister Wilma served as a nurse from 1939 to 1989, working in three hospitals and a rest home in New York and at St. Francis Hospital in Honolulu followed by her assignment at Bishop Home in Kalaupapa. She had three Kalaupapa assignments: her first beginning in the mid 1940s, and her last was a 15-year stretch as supervisory nurse. Sister spent a total of thirty years on Molokai.

In 1988, on her 50th anniversary as a religious, she wrote: "The most important thing which I continue to value is being able to follow in the footsteps of Mother Marianne and Father Damien for more than half of my religious life."

In 1989, Sister returned to Syracuse to minister at St. Francis Social Adult Day Care until she retired to Jolenta Convent, a building adjoined to the Motherhouse.

ADDITIONAL ACKNOWLEDGEMENTS
(see Sr. Wilma's acknowledgements)

After the passing of Sister Wilma, there was an interval of waiting for the book of letters to emerge once again as a worthwhile product to bring to light. Sister Grace Anne Dillenschneider diligently encouraged and worked for its reaching the public. Anwei and Henry Law improved its content by adding photos and working on this effort. Sister Mary Laurence Hanley made the necessary fill-ins and corrections. With the help of Eugene Tiwanek, Sister Alicia Damien Lau chose a printer of exceptional merit. Sister Frances Kowalski received the final approval from the Congregational Leadership Team for the publishing of the *Letters From the Land of Long Farewells*, remarking: "It is a continuation of the legacy of our beloved Mother Marianne Cope and a tribute to her successors."

Table of Contents

Foreword	1
A Song of Farewell	3
Arrival	5
Transportation	17
Daily Routine	25
Kahauko Crater	31
The Dispensary	37
Hunting	43
Night Duty	49
Christmas - Kalaupapa Style	57
New Treatment	63
Dramatics – Kalaupapa Style	77
The Nursery	83
Religious Celebrations	87
Recreation	93
Early Beginnings	99
Molokai	110

Dear Kuuipo in Hawaii and Readers,

I am departing from the accepted form of acknowledgement and writing this in letter form.

I owe a tremendous debt of gratitude to three wonderful people, Sister Eileen Kernan who typed the first copy of these letters and Anwei and Henry Law who did the final work and helped put this together. I type with two fingers. Without these friends, I'd still be typing and you wouldn't be reading these letters.

> With Aloha,
>
> Sr. Wilma

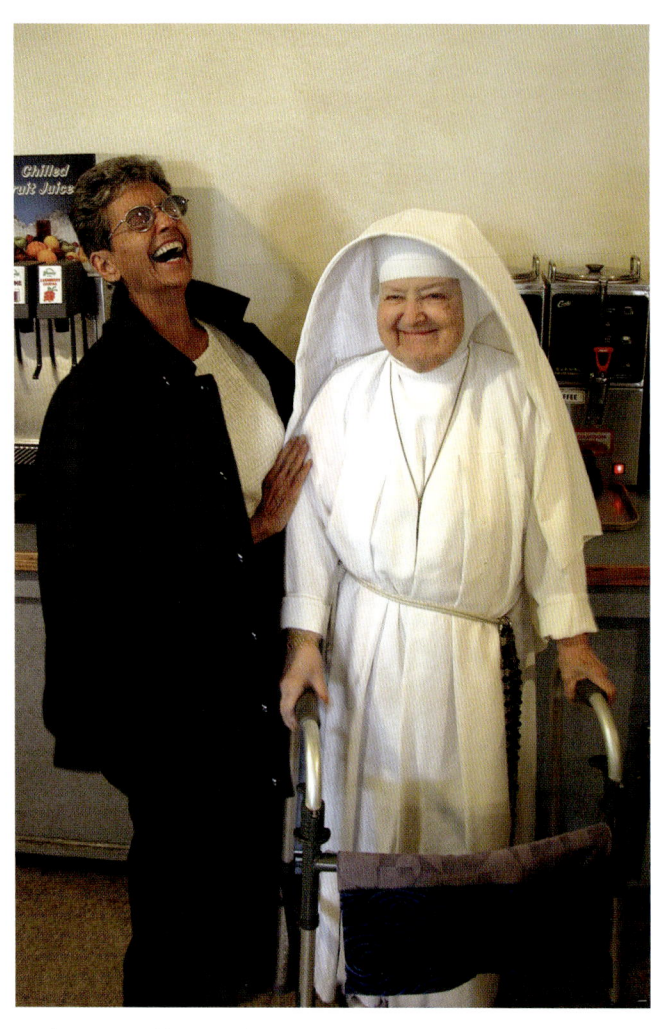

Catching up on old times with Winnie Harada who visited the Motherhouse in Syracuse in 2004. *Photo by Henry Law*

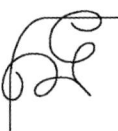

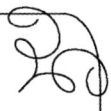

Foreword

These letters were written over fifty years ago, between the years 1946 and the late 1960s. They were put away and forgotten. Recently, they were resurrected.

I have incorporated letters from the records of the Hawaii State Archives to give a sense of the early history of the Settlement. However, the book comprises a record of my early experiences, oral history, and stories told to me by the old residents. I sometimes recount conversations in pidgin English to retain the character of the early residents.

Kalaupapa has come a long way. We carried the torch of Hope in the early days and we didn't hope in vain. The new drugs halted the disease and our people are no longer prisoners. They are allowed to live their lives where and how they wish. More power to them!

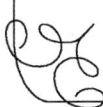

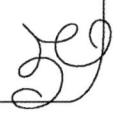

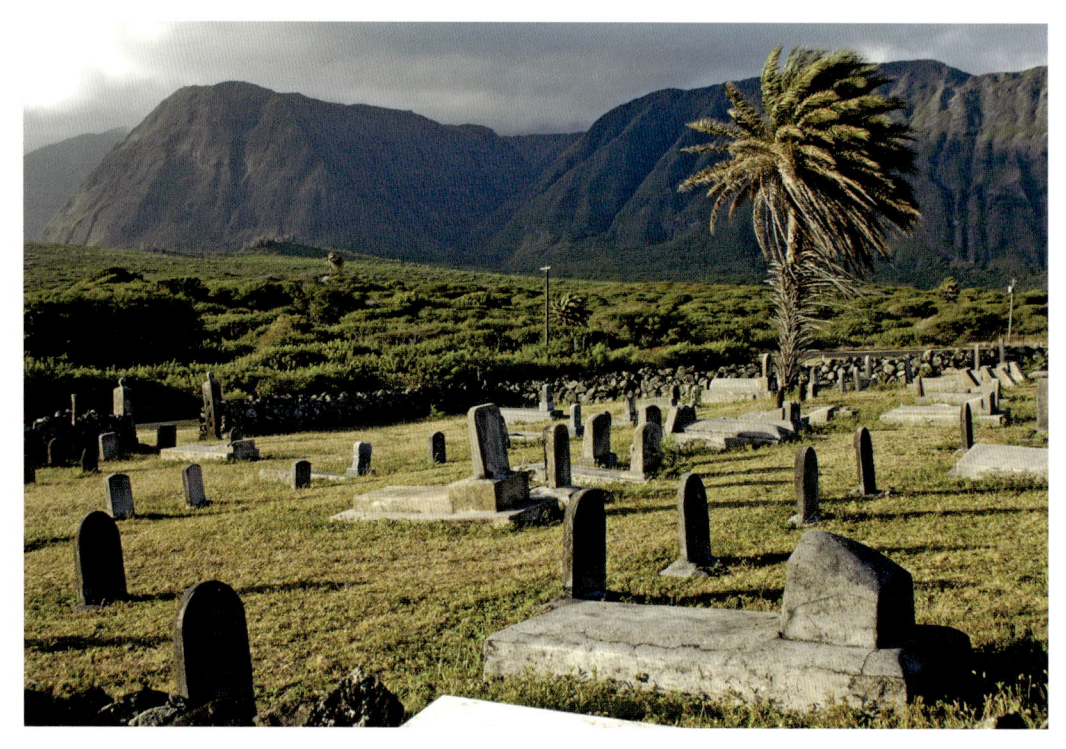

Cemeteries at Kalaupapa reflect the lives of only a handful of the estimated 8,000 people who were forcibly sent to Kalaupapa between 1866 and 1949. *Photo by Henry Law*

A Song of Farewell

The following song of farewell was written by two unidentified Kalaupapa residents in 1922. It gives a real feeling for the great loss experienced by our people when they were taken away from their loved ones and isolated at Kalaupapa because they had leprosy.

Weep no more faithful heart,
Oh! Come no further, here let us part.
Go back home where your kindred still need you
But I need no one.
Beautiful and lost,
All I leave behind,
No dawn awaits me.
Flower of my heart, turn away your eyes.
Try to forget me.

Trees may stand where they grow,
Brooks may harbor the pools they know,
I, alone, am uprooted.
I, who henceforth must be avoided,
Beautiful and lost
All I ever loved
Torn, torn from me.
Flower of my heart
Turn away your eyes,
Try to forget me.
Ah! Try to forget me!
Farewell, farewell.

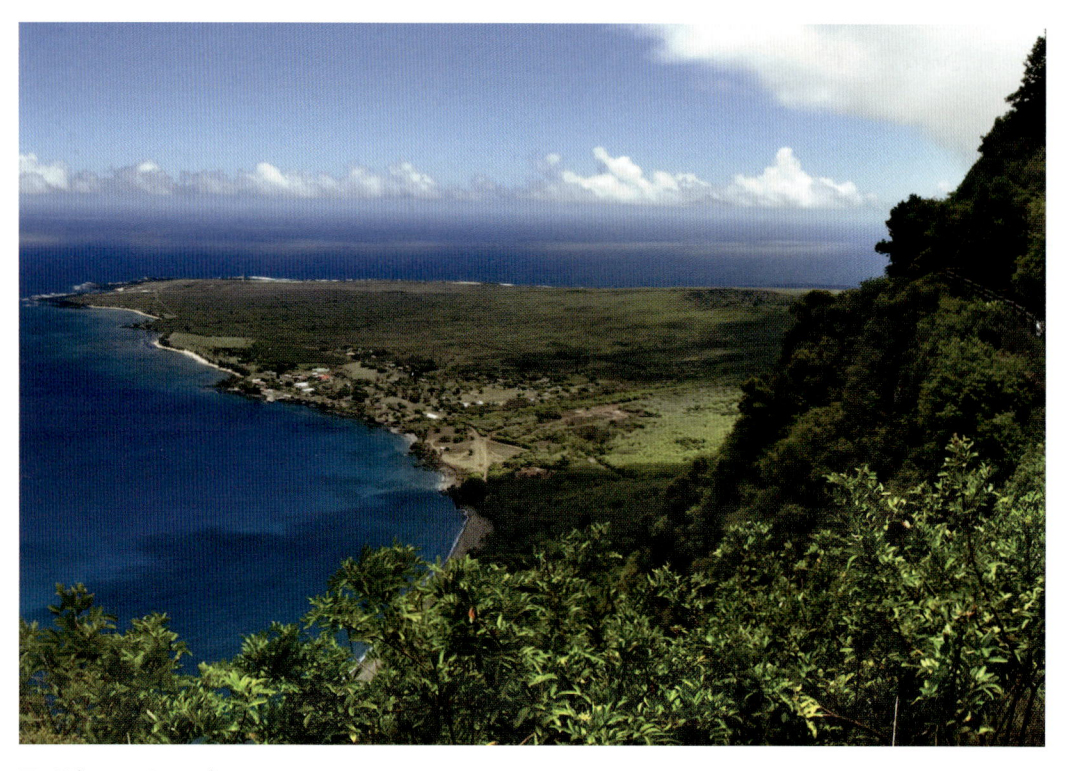

The Kalaupapa Peninsula. *Photo by Henry Law*

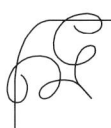

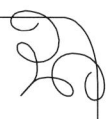

Arrival - 1946

Dear Sister,

Greetings from the island of Molokai! In Hawaiian, Molokai means "Daughter of the Moonlight" and, of course, has a legend attached to it. But you're not interested in legends if I remember correctly.

I can't believe that I'm finally here. When I was in the sixth grade, for an assignment, I read the life of Father Damien. When I finished, I told my family that when I grew up, I was going to Molokai to help Father Damien. Well, here I am 13 years later.

I'm learning to accept centipedes, scorpions, toads, geckos, mongoose, and rats. I should mention the lack of water. Our water supply comes from the valley of Waikolu. Water pipes are laid along the base of the cliffs on a rocky shore. When we have a landslide or high seas, the pipes are crushed and we are without water. If we are lucky and it rains, we gather rainwater in pans and drums. If it doesn't rain, we go to the sea to get what we need.

I arrived in November with three other young nurses to begin work in the Settlement. As we stood on the desolate windswept grass where the plane had deposited us – there is no airstrip, only a meadow -, someone said with a laugh, "We'll probably all meet here again in ten years, but under different circumstances." It was a gloomy thought. Leprosy can have a long incubation period. Before we could become too depressed, we were diverted by the sound of something snorting and laboring up the hill. In a few minutes, a museum piece on four wheels came barreling along at the breakneck speed of about 15 miles an hour. It was the convent car coming to pick us up.

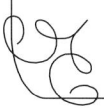

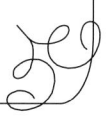

After greeting us, Sister Carmelita squeezed in behind the wheel and prepared for takeoff. "Crawl in where you can," she said.

As we all settled down, I glanced up and asked curiously, "What happened to the roof?"

"Oh, it rotted away. The other day a big chunk fell in and hit Sister Joseph on the head. It's a good thing she has a thick skull."

"What do we do when it rains?"

"We use umbrellas, of course."

I hazarded another question. "What do we do for windows, when it rains, I mean?"

"We use rubber sheets, of course." I could see that living on this island would never be dull.

"Those are some private beach homes," pointed out Sister Mary Joseph as we drove along, "and ahead of us are the cemeteries."

It seemed like an endless stretch of graves along the coastline. Each faith has its own cemetery. We approached a cattle guard which had a large plaque attached to it saying, "WELCOME TO KALAUPAPA."

"Now you are in the town proper," said Sister Mary Joseph.

"The cattle cross the cattleguard on their knees, aren't they intelligent?" said Sister Carmelita with obvious pride.

The village of Kalaupapa is like any other rural village. Many patients have their own homes with lovely yards. There are four churches: Catholic, Protestant, Mormon, and Buddhist. Three have resident clergy. At present, Father Peter is our pastor. There is a Board of Health store where the patients can buy food at wholesale prices. There is also a post office, district court, prison, two large warehouses, a meat house, slaughterhouse, the main office from which all business is transacted, a crematory, bakery, poi shop, laundry shop, gas station, craft shop, theatre, visitors' quarters, and staff quarters.

There are four group homes or compounds: Bishop Home for girls and unmarried women; Baldwin Home for boys and unmarried men, — the Brothers of the Sacred Hearts have charge of it; McVeigh Home for married couples and single persons; and Bay View Home for the more disabled patients. The general hospital has 60 beds for the acutely ill. All other sick people are cared for in the group home infirmaries and by a visiting nurse.

The policies of the Settlement are formulated by the Board of Hospitals and Settlement and all non-patients are civil servants. The patients may also hold jobs if they wish. So, all in all, it is a happy, normal little village.

It was not so in 1866 when the Settlement opened. The King issued an edict in 1865 which would alter the lives of people with leprosy for many years to come. Land was purchased on the remote Kalaupapa peninsula, island of Molokai for segregation of these sick people. They had to build their own shelters because there were only 15-20 houses standing when the land was purchased. Also, what was needed most was a hospital with doctors and nurses to care for the sick. There were only a few medicines entrusted to the superintendent of the Settlement, who was a layman, to dispense at his discretion. Life was a matter of survival of the fittest, and the slogan became, "In this place, there is no law."

This reminds me of a good ghost story.

One day the patients were telling me of the old lady who frequently appears beside the Lang Lang tree on the road to Kalawao. She has been seen for years by our people. Some don't see her but experience a choking sensation when they pass the place. One day one of our patients was out hunting with his dogs. As he drove down the hill, the dogs began to howl and jumped in the front seat which made him swerve. As he skidded past the tree, he saw an old lady with flowing white hair peering at him and pointing a stick at an invisible object across the road. He took a drowning man's grip on the wheel and left the apparition in the dusk.

Another day one of the boys was driving down the hill when suddenly on the road in front of the tree, a huge boulder appeared. He crashed head on into the rock. He knew that this wasn't a natural phenomenon by any stretch of the imagination. He leaped out of the car and ran down the road, not stopping for breath until he got to the village. The road was a good two miles long. The next day the boy went back with friends after having been fortified at Maximo's bar. The smashed car was there but there was no rock to be seen.

I asked the patients if they knew who the lady was. They said that she was an old homesteader who stayed on when the patients came to Kalawao. She had a large comfortable house. The hoodlums of the Settlement wanted the house badly and tried by every means to get it from her, but she fought everyone off. There was nothing left for them to do but kill her. So they made their plans and one day she was ambushed and murdered. That same day the house mysteriously collapsed to the ground and no one profited by her death. To this day, everyone says the lady is still with us.

Meanwhile, all was not totally bad at the Settlement. There still existed Christians who believed in God and continued to gather together whenever they could to hold religious services. The Protestants too formed their little congregation in June of 1866. Several years later, in 1869, they asked the Hawaiian newspaper, The Independent, to publish the following letter for them, asking for help in building their church:

> "In the kindness of your heart, Mr. Editor, will you not do us the favor to telegraph our messages out to all places where Hawaiian People come together? Little by little we have gathered a sum of money to build us a little church . . . . You must not think that all of us here are living in sin and degradation. That is not so. Our greatest longing is to make a memorial to God here . . . . The length of the house we need is 34 feet and its width is 20 feet. It is to have 12 posts in a row. This will cost us as much as $300.00 and will hold a hundred people, for most of us are sick and rarely can more than that number come together. We added up carefully what every one of us could bring to Deacon Muolo. Even with other gifts, it all amounted to $125.00 . . . . The money we have brought together comes from twenty-five cents a week allowed us for extras. We save it bit by bit, though often hungering for the little poi or beef it might purchase at the settlement store . . . . Is there not somewhere among you a good Samaritan? One who will not look at us like the Levite, and pass by on the other side . . ."

What a beautiful testament of faith! The church was built and dedicated in 1871. The Catholic patients also asked friends to help build a house of worship. Four hundred dollars was collected and lumber was purchased for the church. In 1872, Brother Bertrand with a native assistant made the trip to Kalawao with the precious wood and they built the church in six weeks. While Brother Bertrand worked, the patients urged him to ask the bishop for a priest, ". . . because there is plenty of time to die between your visits," and "How are we going to save our souls?" When the church was built, Father Raymond blessed it and named it in honor of St. Philomena. Twelve patients were baptized that same day. The Catholic catechist at that time must have been very zealous because I found an interesting letter among some old documents concerning him or her. I know that we Catholics have been accused of many things, but I must have missed the one about body snatching. Here is the letter.

Kalawao
Molokai
Dec. 25, 1873

To: E. O. Hall
From: S. N. Holokahiki

Abstract
-- Translation in Substance --

The writer states that the Catholic teacher is behaving mischievously, stating that: On the night of December 22nd at about 10:00 p.m., Kaiakoili (K), a member of the Kawaiahao Church, died of leprosy at Kalawao; that the deceased was an ardent believer of Jesus Christ and a faithful member of his church; but at the hour of death, the deceased was baptized stealthily, during the night by Kulia (W) a member of the Catholic Church, without our knowledge.

At dawn the following day, a grave was dug and preparations were made for the burial. The [Protestant] minister . . . . went to Wahinenui, widow of the deceased, and enquired about the hour and place for the memorial services. The widow replied, "The memorial services are to be at the church and burial will be this afternoon." [The] Minister . . . . informed her that he would make preparations and return to conduct memorial services.

In the afternoon he returned, together with friends at the hour agreed upon, to the house of the deceased to conduct the memorial services. Upon nearing the house of the deceased, the minister saw the Catholic teacher standing but removed, in a grumbling manner, mumbling something. At that moment the procession with the coffin proceeded from the house, to the beat of drums. Arriving at the [Protestant] church . . . . the procession did not stop, nor did it enter. The bells of the Catholic Church tolled, and at the Catholic Church the memorial services were conducted by the Catholic teacher.

The writer asks: Are these acts justifiable? Do not these acts constitute thievery? Are not these acts a violation of true justice? The writer believes that the continued residence of the Catholic teacher is unlawful and suggests that the addressee:

    Think the matter over,
    Know the law of prohibiting association
        of non-[patients] with [patients],[1]

---

[1] I have taken the liberty of substituting the word "patient" for the term "leper" in these historic records, but have always indicated the change by putting the word in brackets.

And for that reason believes that the continued residence here
of the Catholic teacher is unlawful.

The writer suggests that Catholics replace said Catholic teacher with a Catholic priest who is also a [patient], and suggesting further that it would be better if a native Hawaiian of that faith were ordained to minister to the members of the Catholic faith.

The people had their wish fulfilled when Father Damien came to stay with them in 1873 and eventually succumbed to the disease, but he was not a Hawaiian. The world knows about the work accomplished by this rough diamond who saw nothing extraordinary about his work. It was something that had to be done and he did it.

There are two stories told to me by the old patients which impressed me very much. Old William, who was an altar boy of Damien's, said that one day when the Settlement was destitute for food, Damien and William swam to the valley of Pelekunu to try to get food. They wore skirts of ti leaves to ward off the sharks. You have to know where Pelekunu is to appreciate what they did. Old William always called Damien "My saint Damien." Another story is that when the patients were shipped to Molokai, they were handcuffed and escorted like criminals to the pier by the police guard. Their families were allowed to accompany them to the pier if they wanted. It happened that the wife of K became a patient and one day she was dragged with other unfortunate people to pier nine to be deported to Molokai. The patient's husband was a giant and possessed incredible strength. When the patients were herded aboard and the weeping and wailing began, he couldn't bear it, so he seized the anchor chain, ripped the holding ring out of the cement and pulled the ship close enough to board. No one stopped him so he went to Molokai with his wife. They say that when he wanted wood, he just pulled a tree up by its roots. Being a good man, he became the champion of the weak in the Settlement. Although he was not a Catholic, he became a good friend of Father Damien and helped him a great deal. One day he confided to Damien that he was afraid of two things. One was that because he was a medical curiosity, the medical profession would get hold of his body after death. The other was that after his death, the Hawaiians would steal his bones to make fish hooks because he was a rarity -- a hairless Hawaiian – and the bones of this kind was needed to make good fish hooks. He made Damien promise that if he died before Damien, that Father would take his body and bury it secretly. Damien promised his friend that he would do so. K died suddenly and Damien secretly buried his body. No one has been able to find it, so K has been able to rest in peace these many years, thanks to his friend Damien.

The following article probably describes the state of the Settlement in the early days fairly accurately. It was written by a Dr. Bechtinger in 1867 for the P.C. Advertiser:

The Leprosy Hospital on Molokai

The great majority of the [patients] are a pitiable sight to behold. I have not seen more than four or five in the whole number who appear to me able to work. The hands and feet appear to be the parts most generally destroyed. How anybody who has seen them should expect them to do much work, I know not. I am satisfied by far that the greater portion of them cannot do much. Their hands and feet are a terrible sight. The disease evidently progresses very rapidly among those who have been sent there. I visited them last April, and on my second visit, I was surprised at the rapid progress of the disease in various individuals. There they are constantly thrown together, in all stages of the disease, with no medicine, no physician, no comforts, furnished with only the absolute necessaries for keeping body and soul together in a well person — and put on starvation rations at that . . . .

The Board of Health has done perhaps as well as they could under the circumstances; but if they cannot control the circumstances better then they are doing now, I shall begin to consider the plan a decided failure. At first, I believed the plan of isolating them there was the best; but having seen how it works, I am more and more inclined to believe the best and least expensive plan would be to have but one hospital, and that in the immediate supervision of the Board of Health and a physician.

The rations for some time past have been four biscuits of hard bread per week to the stronger ones, and ten ditto per week for the feebler ones; and even that, only to those who have been there less than six months. Those who have been there longer are told to work if they want food. Four pounds of salt beef or salmon per week is the allowance of meat to each one.

The beef is a swindle. Much of it is corrupted and some of the barrels are daubed with tar on the inside, which imparts its taste and flavor to the whole contents. The salmon is in good condition. The old thatch houses which were standing when they went there are all the houses they have, except as some of the stronger ones are able to put up huts for themselves. They have no suitable houses for worship and ought to be furnished with a plain frame building for that purpose.

Not withstanding their wretched condition, they have planted some sweet potatoes and other vegetables. They have no kalo [taro] or poi at present, though there is enough kalo land to supply them well, if properly managed. But they have a good quantity of kalo planted, and when it gets ripe, some months hence, may again enjoy their native staff of life. The agent who has immediate charge of them, Mr. Louis Lepart, does as well as he can by them, but is often at his wit's end to know what to do. He can only dole out to them such supplies as he receives from the Board of Health . . . . Many of them have been subsiding in great measure for months past on wild horse-beans, which grow abundantly among the rocks. But the weaker ones cannot endure the fatigue of gathering and roasting them. I am sure, if the Board of Health could see and know the truth in the case, they would endeavor to remedy matters; and yet Mr. Lepart and Mr. Meyers [sic] say they have represented the case to Dr. Hutchingson [sic] . . ."

Slowly, through the years, by dint of much effort, conditions began to change for the better. Today we can lay our weary heads down to rest under a solid roof and on a soft bed, which reminds me that it's time to go to bed. I have to renew my bodily strength so that I can serve God and my brothers and my sisters better tomorrow. A long farewell to you!

With aloha,

Sr. Wilma

Views of Kalaupapa in the 1950's -1960's

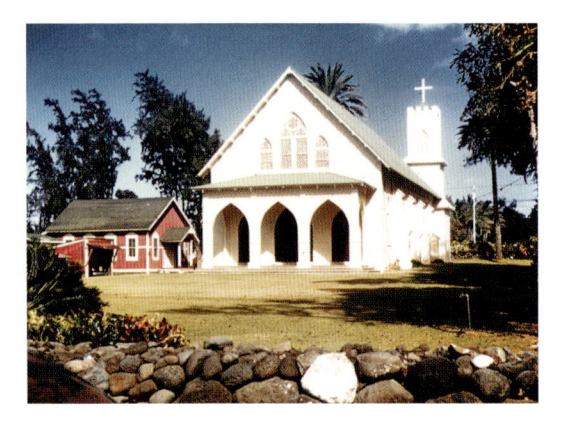

St. Francis Church.

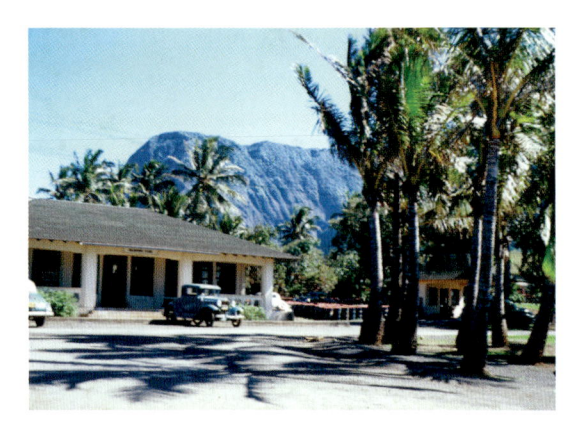

The Board of Health Store which, in the past, was for patients only.

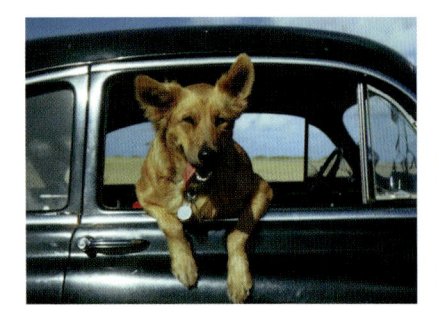

"Happy," our dog.

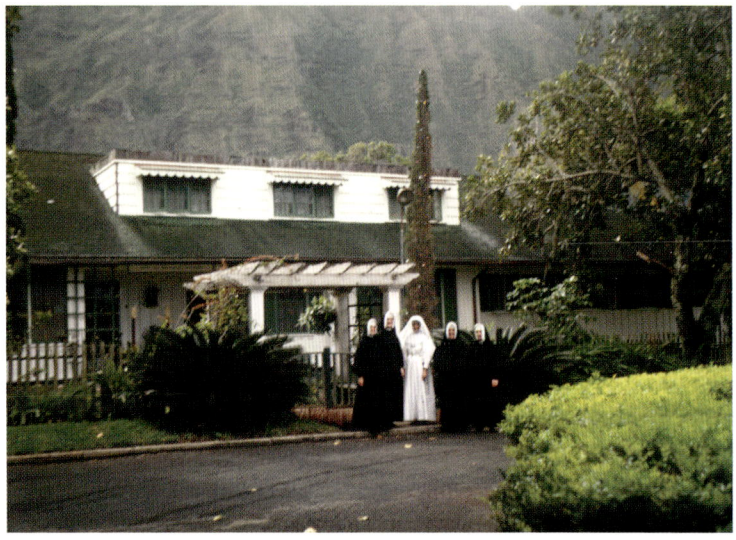

Bishop Home Convent with visitors.

14

Views of Kalaupapa and Kalawao, 2005

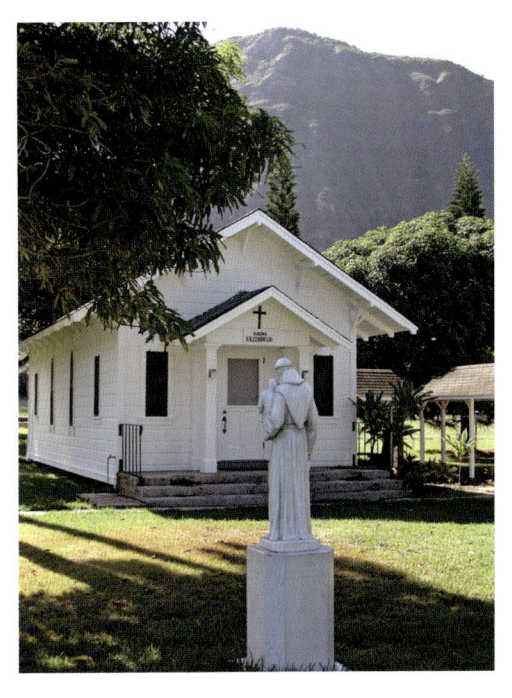

St. Elizabeth Chapel, Bishop Home.

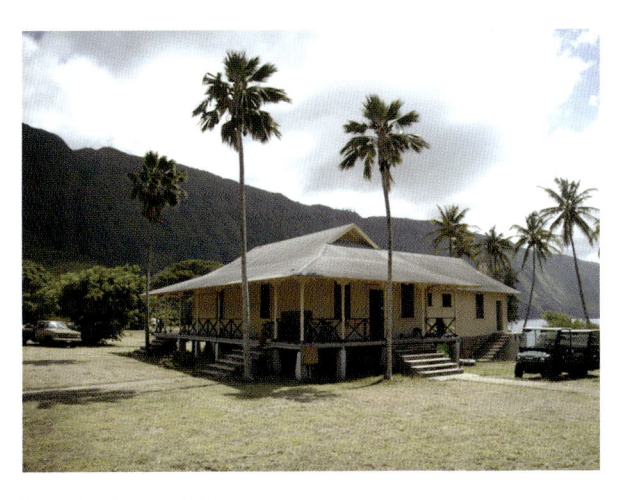

Bay View Home, Kalaupapa.

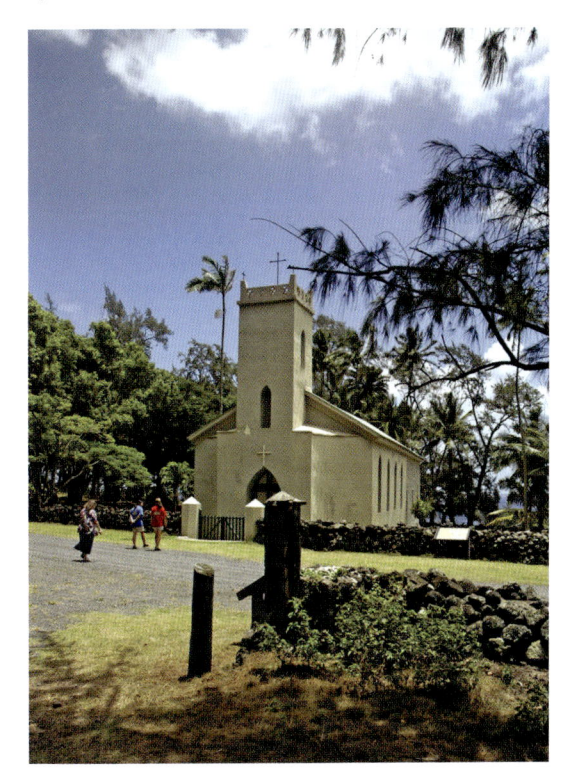

St. Philomena, Father Damien's Church, Kalawao.

Photos this page by Henry Law

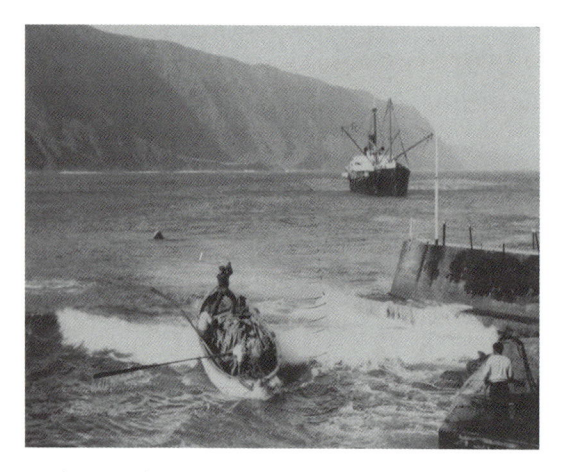

Landing at Kalaupapa, prior to air flights. Almost everyone sent to Kalaupapa initially came by boat.

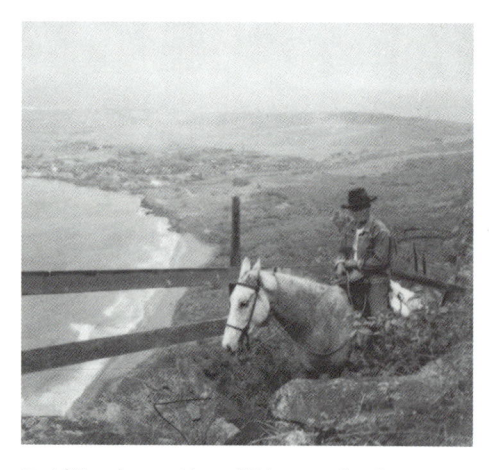

David Kupele, a resident of Kalaupapa for 68 years, carried the mail and movies up and down the trail, sometimes making the trip three times a day.

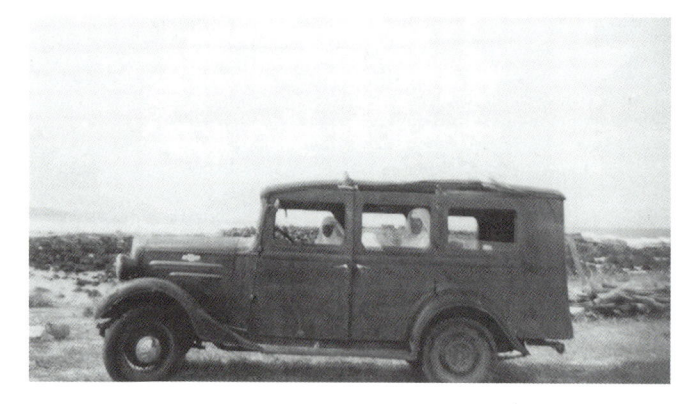

Sisters on an outing.

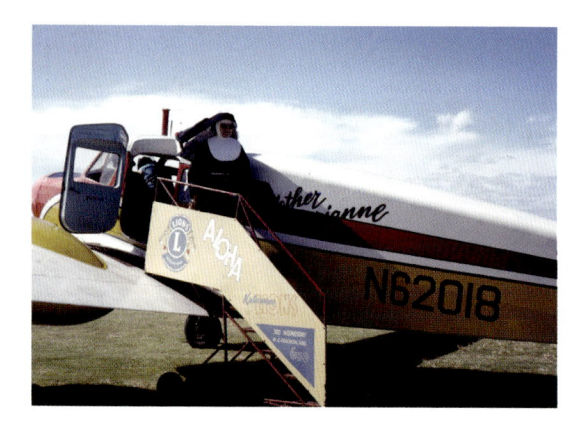

One plane was named after Mother Marianne.

Transportation

Dear Sister,

Here I am again. Since I last wrote to you, I had a strange experience. I touched the top of a rainbow! It happened on the top of our pali (cliff). But I haven't told you about our pali, have I?

When our people were transported to this patch of land many years ago, it was with the idea that they could not escape. They had a choice of jumping into the sea or scaling our two thousand foot cliffs, which wasn't much of a choice. Around this time, a trail was hacked out of the ridge overlooking the ocean. This trail was the Settlement's only link to civilization for a long time, except for the ships which stopped periodically. For years there was at the top of the trail, a gate which was kept locked at all times. The gatekeeper's house was next to it. When we wanted to go up, we had to call, identify ourselves, and say that we had permission to go through. So we were virtually prisoners. All our food, mail, and other necessities were brought down by donkey twice a week, unless bad weather made it impossible. Our muleteer's mule was named "Whiskey." When David couldn't go up, he sent "Whiskey" by herself. She always brought the supplies back safely.

In 1887, Mr. Bishop wrote to his friend, Mr. Meyer, on topside: "I hope it may be necessary for the members of the Board of Health and the doctors to go up and down your pali often, so that something may be done about that road!" He dignified it by calling it a road. It is no more than a goat trail, wide enough for one person. The writer, Charles Warren Stoddard, visited the Settlement and described it very graphically:

> ". . . anon, came steep acclivities with stretches of bare, sun-baked rocks, where our hearts fainted – at least mine did. There was a terrible wall-like cliff that was almost perpendicular; it crumbled as we clung to it like cats, and when I looked below to find my footing, I discovered that the rock upon

which I was stretched in an agony of suspense was apparently overhanging the area, the deep green water was far below me; I felt as if I were climbing into the sky — and then I nearly fell in sheer fright. But a cloud blew over us – they fly low in this latitude; in this thin disguise, I tried to forget that I was suspended in mid air by my eyelids with nothing but sole-leather between me and a thousand feet of space, with certain death at the lower end of it. We were rained upon, shined upon, covered with dust and debris and when we reached the top of the pali, I was dizzy and parched with thirst. It was my last ascent. We made it in two hours and forty minutes, with my heart knocking at my ribs all the way up. It is truly the mountain of difficulty."

A few days ago, Sister Claudia and I went up the trail because we felt in need of exercise. I used an umbrella for a walking stick. When we were almost at the top, a rain cloud descended on us and gave us a drenching. I put the umbrella up but it promptly blew inside out and sailed over the cliffs. Then the rainbow appeared below us. It was so lovely that I had to reach out to touch it. We sat on a rock and ate our sandwiches while we watched the rainbow glide over the Settlement --- a sign of God's blessing.

We haven't used the trail for transporting supplies since 1950 when our airstrip was finished. It's a short runway – we tried to enlarge it, but when the men removed a certain rock which was in the way, the rock came back to its original position. This happened again and again. The men reported it to the administrator of the Settlement who was a Hawaiian. He looked at the rock and said that it was part of a heiau [Hawaiian place of workship] and to leave it alone. So the air-strip was not enlarged.

The day for the official opening of the runway dawned bright and beautiful, and everyone who was able, went down to see the grand opening. "Here comes the plane!" someone shouted.

"Where?" We were all shielding our eyes from the blinding sun.

"Over the pali." We watched the Andrews plane curve gracefully over the water and straighten out for the landing. Before we knew what happened, the plane crash-landed on the runway. To make a long story short, a wild time was had by all.

It is a wonderful experience to fly in one of these freight planes which are small two engine Cessnas. We call them paper planes, which is misleading to the novice traveler. They are not made of paper as some suppose, but carry our daily newspaper among other things. The plane is first loaded with the freight and then passengers get in where they can.

It is a very informal situation. The last time I flew from Honolulu, the pilot said, "Get in, Sister."

I looked into the plane and said, "Where?"

"Just crawl over the papers into the co-pilot's seat."

Being conditioned to obedience, I crawled in on hands and knees, got my posterior stuck and had to flatten myself on my stomach to crawl forward. I had to go into the seat head first. You have to throw decorum to the wind sometimes. Of course, it is better to have the plane full, because when it is emptier, it shakes and bounces as though it were in the throes of a St. Vitas dance.

I'll describe one of my recent trips from Honolulu to Molokai to give you an idea of what it is like. "I'm sorry, but the weather isn't the best for flying today, but I have to get back to Kalaupapa." I get into the plane and position myself in the pilot's seat. Herman, our pilot, looks over and grins at me. He knows how I hate to fly.

"Okay, Sister, then fasten your seat belt." The motors cough and sputter as Herman tries to get the propellers started. One motor won't turn over and

Herman frowns. To see Herman frown spells disaster to me because he always reminds me of those deodorant ads: always cool and calm, no sweat. The motor gives a desperate cough and starts up sluggishly and we begin to taxi to the runway, which is quite a distance off. We are fourth in line for a take-off. WHOOSH!

We just got the backfire of a BOAC rushing by and our little plane rocks like a cork on a rough sea. I keep mopping my brow because there is no air conditioning. WHOOSH! Another backfire. Relax, we won't turn a somersault, but I'm glad that I didn't eat any lunch before I left. The earphones crackle with a lot of unintelligible gibberish, but Herman doesn't look worried so it must be OK. Finally we get in position for the take off.

"Is your seat belt fastened, Sister?" I mutely nod in the affirmative. Since we got into position, I've made the sign of the cross and clenched my teeth in preparation. The motors roar deafeningly and the plane strains at its leash like a nervous race horse. Herman looks over the panel. It must be OK because he looks calm. Suddenly the runway rushes at us. I've said a prayer to St. Michael, St. Christopher, and our Lady of the Airways and there isn't much runway left. I dig my heels into the floor in readiness for a crash. Our load must be too heavy. Finally we lift a little and the Mother Marianne is airborne. Thank God! Mr. Andrews named two of his planes Mother Marianne and Father Damien.

"It's going to be a little rough," Herman informs me.

We fly through a huge cloud formation and are suddenly in a fairyland. The plane bounces around in the air currents, but I'm busy building castles out of the clouds. WHOOSH! – I strain against my seat belt as I shoot upward. We just hit an air pocket and my stomach flies up into my mouth as I quickly clamp my teeth together. I settle down. As I move my feet, my long habit suddenly flies over my face. When I disentangle myself, I look down. I see a hole in the floor which must have been covered with my feet. I can actually see the water below us. Suddenly, I don't hear the motors! I swallow in panic and find to my relief that my ears were plugged only from the pressure. I'm relaxing when Herman gives me a jab with his elbow which sends me straight up. This must be it! Get ready to bail out! When I assemble my scattered wits, I see that Herman is pointing to something below, and there is a whale spouting a fountain of water. A lovely sight. Suddenly a red light shows up on the panel. "What's that?" I ask in alarm.

"One gas tank is empty," Herman informs me. So I start another rosary. Molokai is completely hidden by heavy clouds. We should be over or near Molokai since we've been in the air over twenty minutes. We keep flying in a circle looking for land. Suddenly there is a small break in the clouds and Herman, seeing land, dives down like a homing pigeon before he loses sight of it. Our runway is so long, that if you sneeze, you can overshoot it, but Herman puts the Mother Marianne down, bouncing and skidding. Fortunately, we are in one piece. Thank God for great favors! Herman fills the empty tank and takes off again while I pray for his safe return.

In the old days, if people wished to enter the Settlement, they came by boat and landed at Kalaupapa. The ship anchored a good way from our shore, and the people came in by rowboat. One climbed down a rope ladder, and the trick was to jump when the boat came up on a wave. Over the years, several of the boats capsized and some people were lost.

We have some very bad weather at times. This reminds me of a good story:

The Kaala was a ship that brought freight to the various islands. On this occasion, it was bringing badly needed supplies to Kalaupapa. I'll give you the newspaper version and then the real McCoy.

1940 — Sampan Hits Molokai Reef in Whirlwind

The sixty-five foot sampan Kaala, used by the territorial Board of Hospitals and Settlement to transport supplies to the Kalaupapa Settlement on Molokai, ran aground off Kalaupapa Friday night.

The boat was caught in a freak whirlwind during the rainstorm and was flung onto the reef close to the shore. The four crew members are reported safe, but the Kaala and its twenty-five ton cargo are believed to be a complete loss according to Harry Kluegel, general superintendent of the Board of Hospitals and Settlement. Mr. Kluegel said the sampan was carrying medical supplies and equipment seriously needed by the Kalaupapa residents . . .

One of the crewmen on the ship later became a patient and told me the real story. Here it is: During the evening the people of the Settlement heard the frantic blasts from the Kaala's horn and ran down to the pier to investigate. There was no Kaala in sight. Finally they saw her floundering on a reef, way off course. No one could figure out how it landed where it did. The true story is that all on board were drinking and the captain mistook the lighthouse beam for the light on the landing pier, and set course accordingly. The lighthouse stands on a hill far inland. Naturally, the ship ran aground. A rusty piece of the ship can still be seen rising out of the water, its nose pointed toward the fatal beam. So much for newspapers!

I hope this short letter finds you in the best of health. I'll write again soon.

With Aloha,

Sr. Wilma

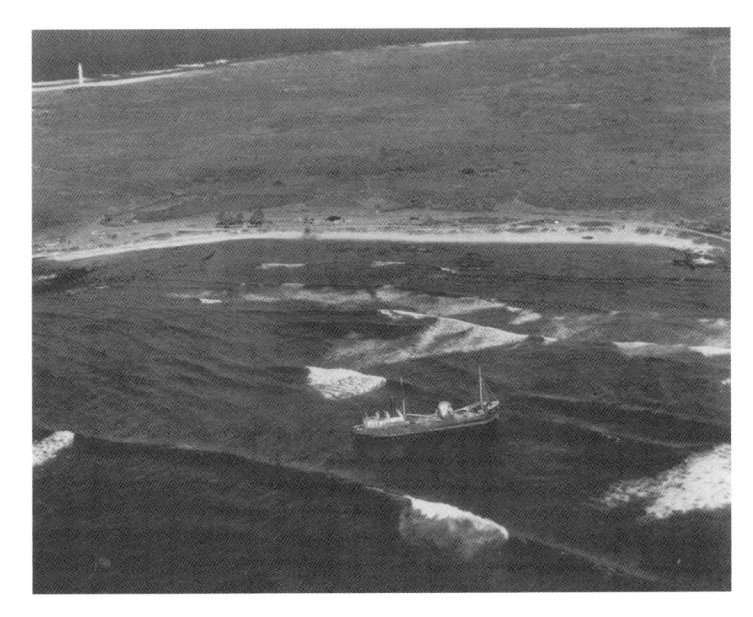

The S.S. Kaala on the rocks at Kalaupapa. Courtesy IDEA

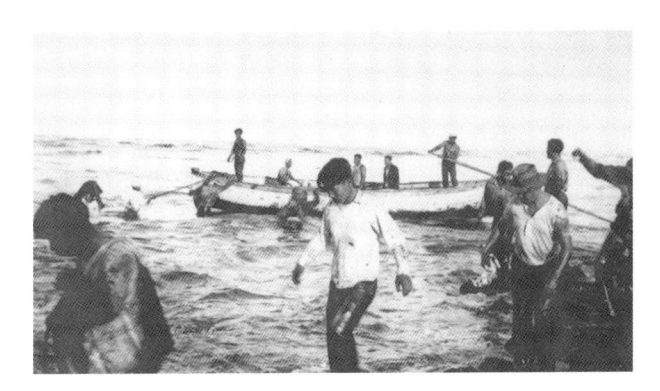

Crew of the Kaala come ashore.

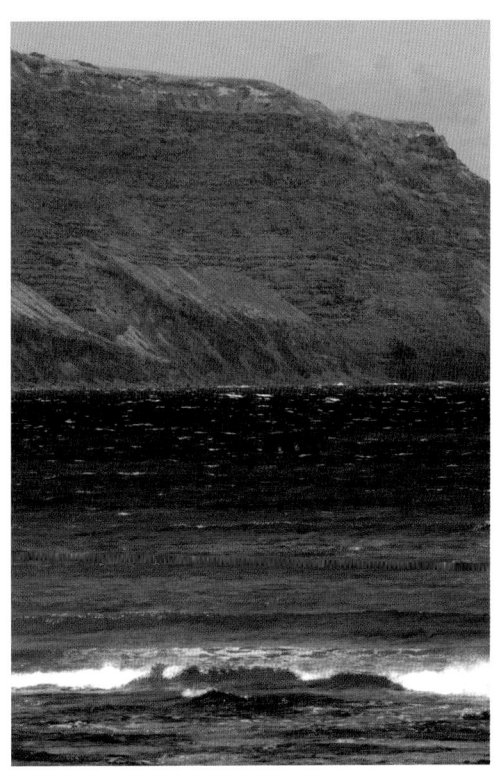

All that can be seen of the Kaala today. *Photo by Henry Law*

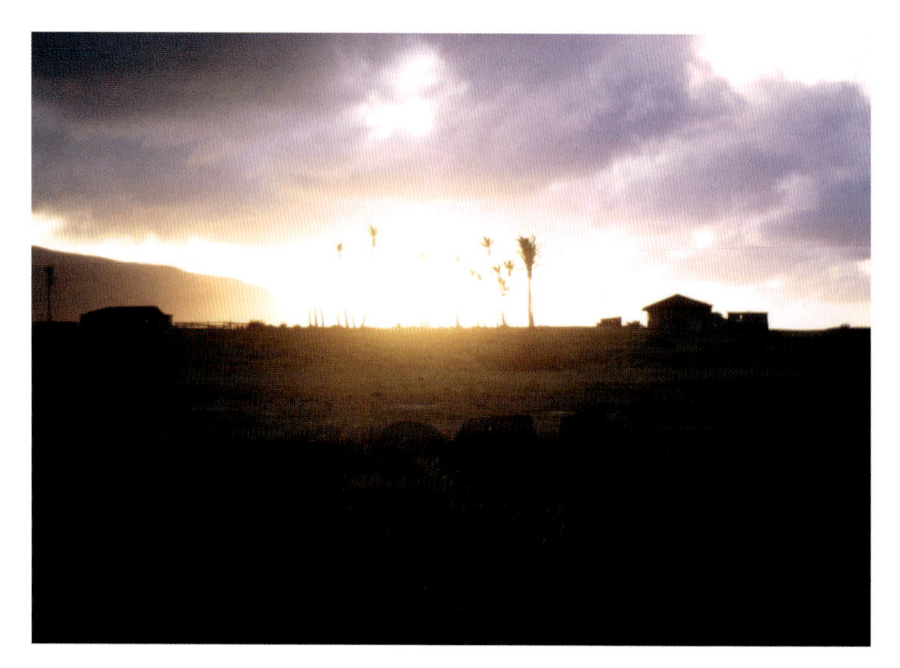

Sunset over the beach houses at Kalaupapa.

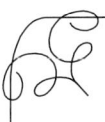

Daily Routine

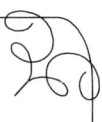

Dear Sister,

The shades of evening are gently descending on another day as I write this, and we are one day closer to eternity. Time seems to fly on the wings of the wind on Molokai.

You asked how our days are spent here. My dear, not one of them is ever dull, and each one seems to be more challenging than the day before. The healthy combination of love of God and challenge keeps us going.

I must begin by saying that our superior has a mania for being on time. Consequently, we put the convent clock 15 minutes ahead. So we rise with the neighbor's rooster. It sometimes happens that we rise ahead of him. For some reason, this annoys me no end. On rising, I say that lovely prayer:

> Good morning, God, and thank You for
> The glory of the sun.
> And thank You for the health I have
> To get my duties done.
> I will devote the hours of
> This golden day to You,
> To honor Your most Holy Name
> In everything I do.

I'm careful to shake out my clothes before I dress and check my shoes for centipedes and scorpions. I chalk this up to experience.

The walk from the house to chapel at that time of morning is so refreshing and the stars are still visible. It reminds me of an old Indian proverb:

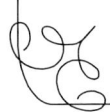

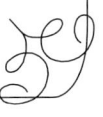

> "However my eyes may wander, Thou standeth before me.
> For the heavens and the splendor of the stars are Thy image."

This is a lonely place. In the early morning, as we kneel in chapel in meditation, the only sound to be heard is the plaintive call of the mourning dove far across the plains. There are no large buildings to impede its path. We go to the parish church of St. Francis at 5:50 a.m. for Mass, and we begin our work at 7:00 at the hospital. We finish at 5:00 in the afternoon.

Of course we are on call 24 hours a day for emergencies. It's a long day. The sulfone drugs are just being introduced and everyone is not on them yet, so we still have heavy cases. The hospital has 60 beds which are filled with very sick patients. The other bed patients are cared for in each unit (group) home infirmary. If they become acutely ill and there is room in the hospital, they come to us. The physician makes daily rounds to all the Homes.

There are six wards in the hospital, two of which are T.B. wards. Surgery, Lab, X-ray, Dental, and ENT are kept busy with both in-patients and out-patients. In the out-patient department, there is a constant stream of patients from 7:00 a.m. to noon for dressings, ENT, dental, and changing of tracheotomy tubes. Our medical director says that most Lepromatous patients who live long enough develop laryngeal stenosis in time and require a tracheotomy. At present we average between 7-16 people a year who require this operation.

With the advent of the sulfones, we hope for a brighter future for our patients. It's a little nerve wracking to watch a patient with a choking spell. Recently, one of our new trachea patients who was having trouble jumped out of bed and tried to push a large pair of scissors down the tube in a desperate attempt to get air. It was lucky that I had just gone in to check on her. Another patient died coughing up bits of his trachea. It took days. As he coughed up the cartilage, we pulled it out with forceps to keep him from choking. He was such an edifying patient. He never complained and he knew that he was dying. He willed his clock to the

Sisters, and asked us to put it in chapel so that when we looked at it, we would say a prayer for his soul. I'm sure that he is praying for us in Heaven.

The nurse is on duty from 5:00 p.m. to 7:00 a.m. alone. Up until 11:00 p.m. she has two orderlies to help her to empty bed pans, give nourishment, and change incontinent patients. After that she is alone until 5:00 a.m.

One night a funny thing happened to me on the way to the morgue. I was taking a patient there. One of our patients had a series of choking spells and apparently died. Being very busy, I couldn't take him to the morgue immediately. A few hours later, I was hurrying down with my burden when suddenly the shrouded figure moved. I almost fainted. I summoned up courage to snatch off the sheet – and glory be to God – he was breathing. So I rushed him back to bed before he realized where he was going.

Did I tell you what our morgue looks like? Well, there is a little stone building next to the hospital. One side is the morgue and the other is the mental room we use for psychiatric patients. In the morgue there are only three small windows for ventilation. The room feels like a sweat box. I'll say nothing of the smell. The autopsy table is made of masonite, not steel, and is in the shape of a V, not flat. The V acts as a trough. There is a small hole in the middle to catch the fluid, and we place a bucket under it for the fluid. Then we have a small sink where we wash the organs. Then, don't be shocked, they think that I am too fastidious when I raise my voice in outraged protest, we use a butcher knife from the kitchen to cut up the specimens and the kitchen scales to weigh the organs. "What's the difference," they say. "Everything is washed off, isn't it?" Perhaps in time, I too will become hardened, but every time I assist, my stomach is rocky for a few days. When one reads the autopsy reports, one wonders how our people were able to stand on their feet for so long.

When we are on day duty, we do one month of dressings in the wards, then one month of float, which means that we do all the treatments, give medications, and all the nursing care. Two nurses are assigned to dressings and treatments in the out-patient department. One is assigned to I.V. therapy. Blood transfusions are given weekly to patients with extremely low hemoglobin.

When a patient dies, the nurse on duty prepares the body for burial and puts it in the coffin because we do not embalm here. The people tell me that until about ten years ago, the coffin makers made their rounds in the hospital every day to ascertain who was eligible for a coffin and would measure them for one.

I am glad that this custom has been done away with. So you can see by this epistle that our days are quite full but we still manage to enjoy the beauty which surrounds us and try like Hildegard to be "a feather on the breath of God," allowing God to blow where He wills.

With Aloha,

Sr. Wilma

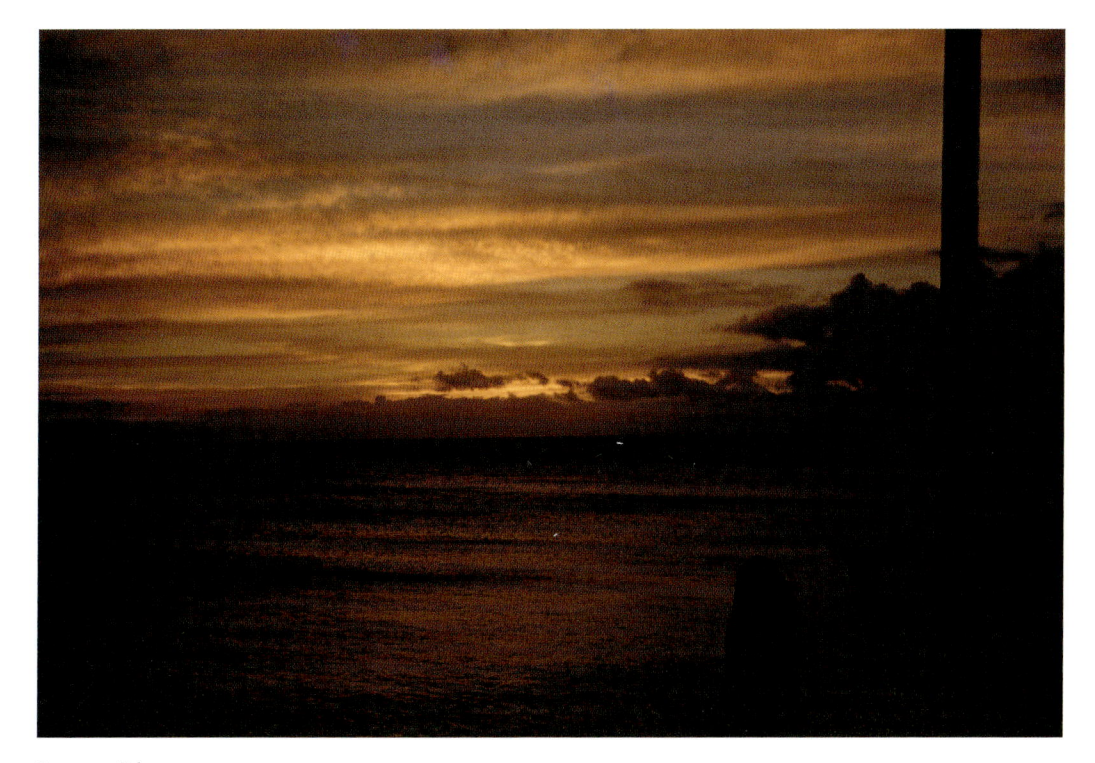

Sunset at Kalaupapa.

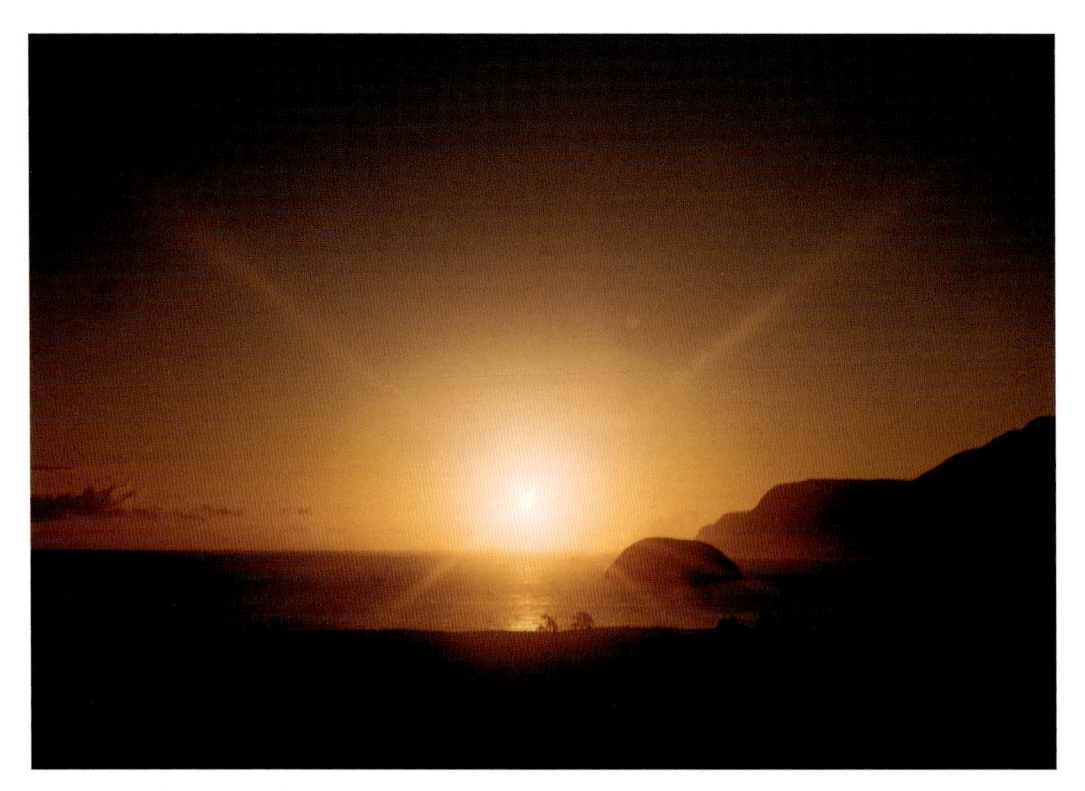

Sunrise over Kalawao as seen from the crater.

*Arise lyre and harp
With praise let us
awake the dawn.*

Kauhako Crater

Dear Sister,

I think that you would be interested in hearing about our crater. When one thinks of it, we are rather unique. Our peninsula is only a little over three miles long and we have a crater in the center of it. Thank God that it is extinct.

The island of Molokai was at one time two pieces of land which later fused together. One side is a series of beautiful mountains and valleys and the other side is all flat land. A long time later, the vent for the subterranean forces which formed our peninsula and attached it to the larger island became known as Kauhako Crater. The land was divided into three sections.

Kalawao means "hog" or "robe." It was thought that the land received this name because the ancient dwellers were annually taxed a hog or a dress by the reigning chiefs.

The eastern portion was named Kalaupapa or the leafy plain or flat.

The middle portion was named Makanalua or "the given grave or pit" because in ancient times the lake at the bottom of the crater was used as a burial ground for the dead. It was considered a good omen if the body sank because this was proof that the soul was accepted into the spirit world. If the corpse floated, then – Auwe! It was a pilau sign! The simple explanation is that the lake which covers some five thousand square feet is composed of brackish water. It is the apex of a funnel which ends in the sea. At low tide, a large amount of fresh water enters the lake from the far off basin of Waihanau Falls in the valley of Waihanau. This fresh water floats on top of the underlying sea water. The tides and not the spirits determine whether the bodies sink or float.

Some of our old timers told me that in later years the bodies were tied to a plank and were carried down to a cave whose mouth was situated below the water and were deposited there. I asked if the cave was wet, and they said no that it was a dry cave. They say that there are many bodies buried there. No wonder it is believed that the spirits roam the floor of the crater at night.

The ancient Hawaiians used the floor of the crater as one of their worshiping places so there must be a heiau there somewhere.

A heiau is an altar of sacrifice. There are several types. The Ka'a could be built by the common people and placed in the home if desired, but generally heiaus were built along the seashore. We have our share of them in Kalaupapa. The offerings on these heiaus were bananas and pigs.

The Waihau could only be built by chiefs. Offerings here were coconuts, bananas and hogs.

The Luakini could only be built by a king. Before this type could be consecrated, human sacrifice had to be offered. After this was done, it was called the heiau pookanaka or temple of sacrifice. We had two of these heiaus of which I am aware: Kakuiopuu, which is situated high on the Kalaupapa cliffs and measures 100 feet x 60 feet, and Puuakahi, which was situated at the base of our present pali.

There is an interesting story told about this heiau: In ancient times, the chiefs of the other islands liked to come to Kalaupapa for surfing and relaxation. Lanoikahakahiki moi of Hawaii set out with his wife and a large retinue to look for wood on the island of Kauai, suitable for the making of spears. The party decided to land at Kalaupapa for rest and refreshment. Lanoikahakahiki settled down to play a game of kamana or Hawaiian checkers. The people were very fond of playing this game. His wife in the meantime went off with her lover, who was a young man in the king's retinue. The checker game was suddenly and rudely interrupted when a loud voice trumpeted from the heiau, "Lanoikahakahiki, your wife betrays you with Hea Kakoa."

"Auwe!" The king jumped up in a rage and seizing the checker board — not an easy feat because they are made of a large stone slab — went looking for his wife. When he found her, he smashed the board over her head. Notice, he didn't do anything to the man. Amazingly, the wife didn't die but followed Lanoikahakahiki to Kauai. Poor soul!

Now the Hawaiians have what is called Aikua, the 14th night of the moon, or the dark night of the moon, when it is believed the night marchers walk the earth. They are believed to be the spirits of the dead kings and warriors and supposedly the ancient gods. The night of Kane is the night when the kings and their retinue walk. In Kalaupapa, the land is unspoiled by human progress, and the spirits of the dead are rumored to roam about very freely. So on the night of Kane, our people speak about seeing the marchers. These marchers consist of Keawe, known as the headless king, and his retinue. They carry their burial equipment with them. The Alii (royalty) carry their canoes and the lesser folk carry their tapa mats rolled neatly under their arms. Some Hawaiians claim that they have heard the flutes and drums and also the chanting and the bark of dogs. The procession reportably begins at the site of the heiau Puuakaha. When it reaches Bishop Home, the people stop behind our infirmary to rest before going on to the crater. The Hawaiians say that if you see the procession coming, you must get out of the way or it will mean certain death for you.

But to get back to the crater, some of us have been fascinated by Kauhako, and we decided to go down into it and explore it, if possible. I enquired around to ascertain if there were trails leading to the lake which is located in the crater's center. From the mauka side, the wall is straight down. If you are afraid of heights, it's a good place to stay away from.

From reliable sources, we heard that yes, there was a good trail made recently, a few years ago, and that it was easy to get down. So one fine day, six of us started down. The trail is negotiable if you are fortunate to wear AA shoes for there is only room for one foot. To further complicate matters, the negotiable part of the trail is covered with iron wood needles, which makes the trail like a sheet of ice. I zoomed down part of the way like a flailing windmill, with an arm and a leg flapping over the void to keep my balance. It was a memorable experience. I couldn't even say an act of contrition.

We finally got to a place which seemed straight down and I refused to budge. Our guide, who seems to be part mountain goat, insisted that the trail gets better as we go down. So I sat on a boulder and waved my legs around trying to find something to step on. There was nothing but air. Finally by sliding down a little farther and stretching myself as far as possible, I felt a rock under my feet and I let go. Simultaneously, the rock gave way and we went down together. I snatched at a branch of a stout tree as I flew by, but the tree was dead and it came with me. I was still clutching the wood when I landed.

The floor of the crater is like a jungle. We hacked our way through the heavy vines and century plants with a machete. Suddenly we found ourselves looking over another rim into the water. This side of the rim was straight down about 50 feet. The other side is sloping, but still very steep.

One of the Sisters found a tree that wasn't dead and she tied a rope to it. This is the only way of getting down without falling in. Wanting to get a better look, the doctor with us stepped forward – unfortunately onto a wet piece of foliage. His feet shot from under him and down he zoomed. As he went by the Sister clutching the tree, she thought of grabbing him by the trousers. Then she thought it wouldn't be proper and hoped he could swim. Fortunately, he was stopped by a huge cactus plant. With the help of the rope, he climbed back. Everything considered, a good time was had by all. On the way back, when we got to the slippery part of the trail, I had to go up on my hands and knees. I vowed that if I got back in one piece, I would never go back again. Perhaps, when you come over to visit, we can take you down. Keep well and God bless you.

With Aloha,

Sr. Wilma

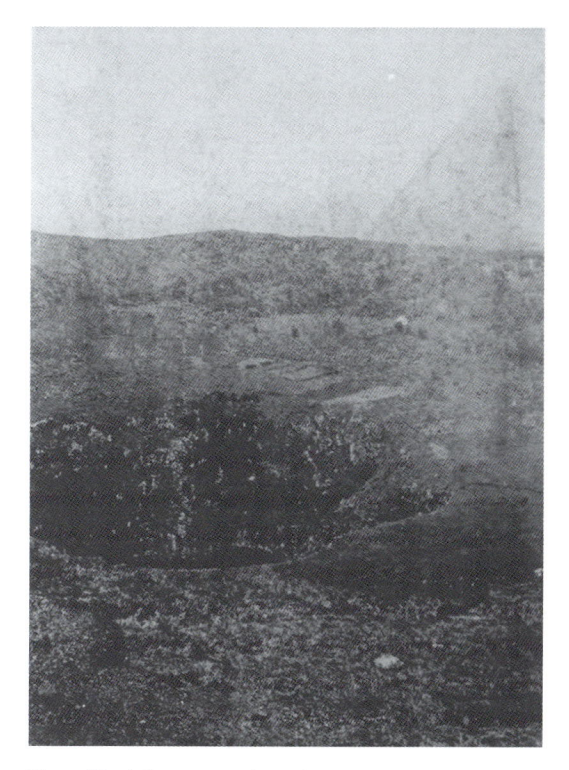

View of Kauhako crater in the early times.

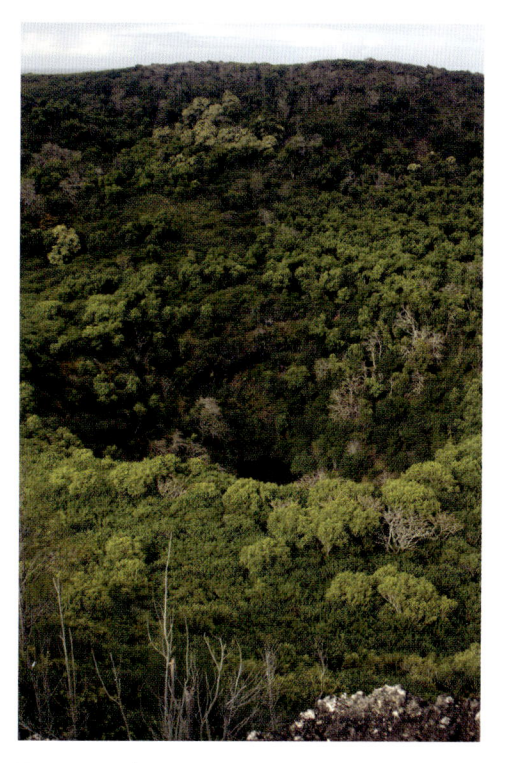

The crater today. *Photo by Henry Law*

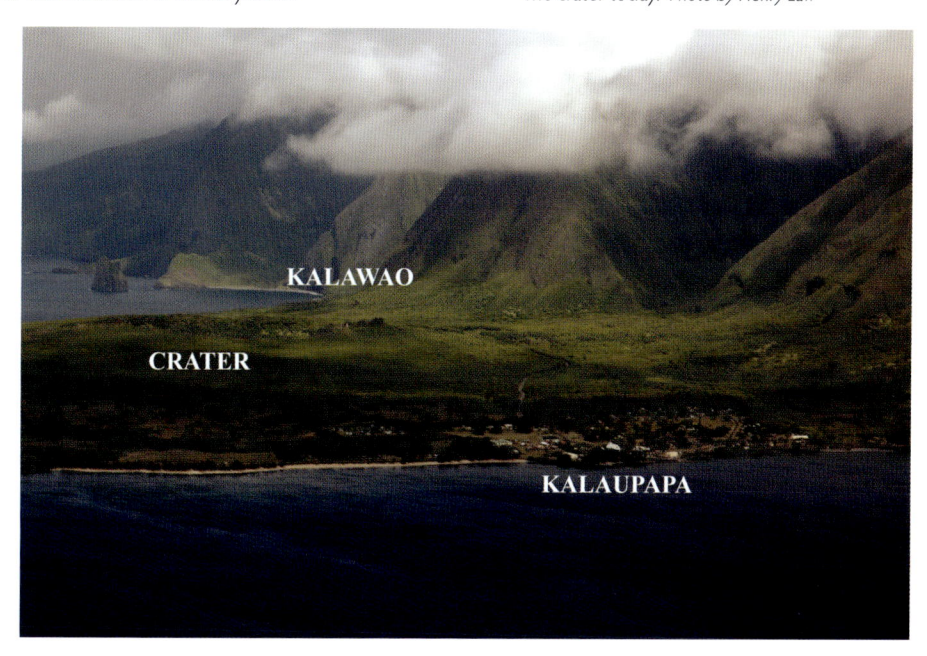

The Kalaupapa Peninsula, showing the location of the crater. *Photo by Henry Law*

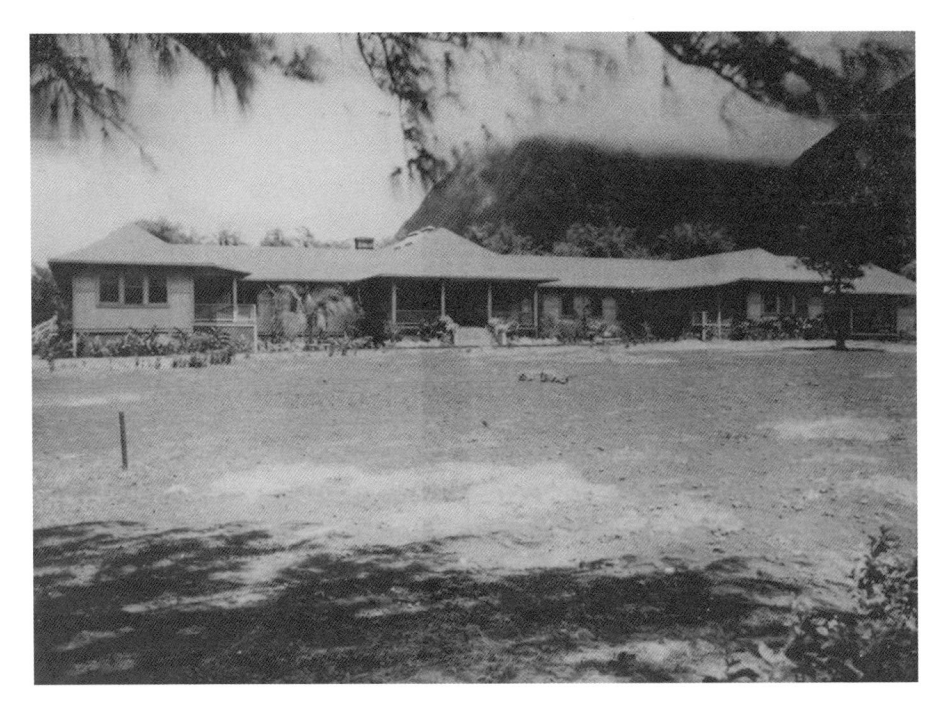

The old Kalaupapa Hospital, built in 1932

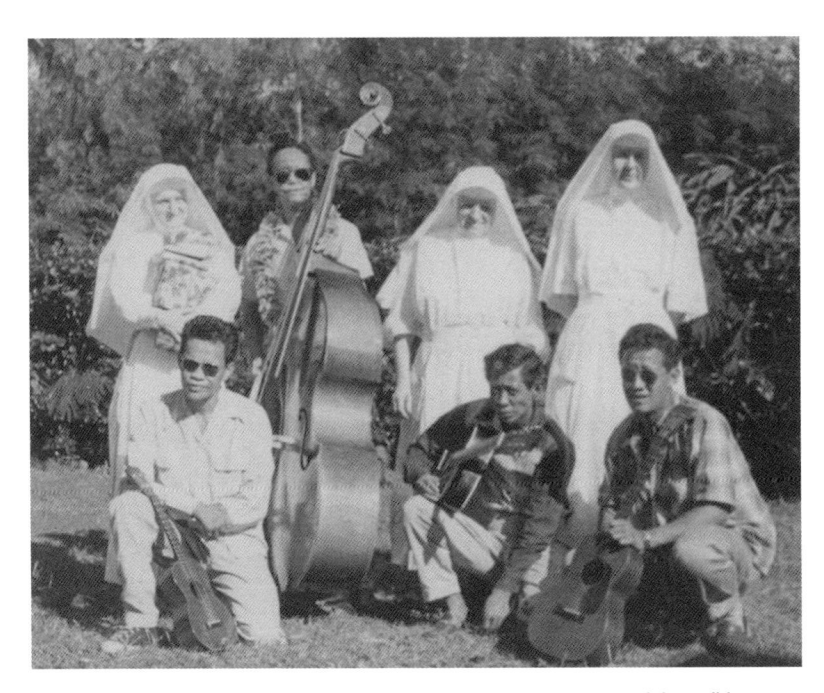

Sisters with Kalaupapa musicians. Sammy Kuahine, with the bass, composed the well-known song, "Sunset of Kalaupapa."

The Dispensary

Dear Sister,

This month I am assigned to the dispensary in the out-patient department. I enjoy this very much although the work is hard. We work full speed from 7:00 a.m. to noon. We see half of the Settlement in the course of the morning in spite of the fact that we have a visiting nurse making rounds.

In the dispensary, we change and sterilize the trachea tubes of all the patients. Each tube is different in size and shape, so we have to be very careful not to mix them up. We give ear, nose, and eye treatments plus dressings of ulcers. These ulcers vary in size and severity. Some are deep enough to expose bone and are malodorous. There is a kind which we unscientifically call "the termite kind" because it begins at one spot, then tunnels its way along the flesh, leaving ribbons of flesh on the body. It is extremely painful. I had one patient, who when she died, was one mass of ribboned flesh. We couldn't find a spot to give her an injection. In the dispensary also, the nurse removes sequestra or degenerative bone from the hands and the feet. This would be called minor surgery elsewhere, but here it is a nursing procedure.

In spite of their numerous afflictions, our people are a happy people. The younger generation bring their ukeleles and guitars to the hospital and, while they wait, they play and sing many of the lovely Hawaiian songs. In this department, everything is discussed from theology to politics and the more scandalous secrets of the moment. After a few weeks in this department, one acquires quite an education.

One day we began by talking theology of a sort. "Red" began by saying that God was a working God and that when we went to heaven, we would have to work for all eternity because we had to follow God's example. This started quite a discussion which I abruptly ended by saying, "Well, Red, I'm knocking myself out working down here and I intend to play the harp when I get up there."

"How can you say that, Sister? If God works, then you have to work also."

"I'll tell you what, Red. Every morning when you walk past my window on the way to work, I'll give a few plucks on my harp to cheer you along."

If looks could kill, I'd be dead. From this discussion we shifted to the subject of spirits, and how they roam the world, especially Kalaupapa. I laughed, and Red who was still chafing said, "You better be careful, Sister, some day you'll laugh out of the other side of your mouth." For once, he was right.

"Have you heard about the Lizard Lady?" someone asked. "I've heard of Lorelei, but I must have missed the one about the lizard."

There are many stories about the Lady who lives in the basin of water at the foot of the falls in Waihanau, but I will repeat one.

One night, it was a time when the Baldwin Home for Boys was still in Kalawao; the boys were walking home from the movies which were shown in Kalaupapa; One has to pass Kauhako Crater and Waihanau Valley on the way to Kalawao. The boys were walking along laughing and talking when they saw Ramon, who was bringing up the rear, veer off and begin to walk toward the mouth of the valley. The other boys thought that it was strange but they did nothing about it. When the group finally settled down for sleep and Ramon hadn't yet shown up, the boys began to get worried. Some of them went to the Brother in charge to report what had happened.

"We better go back and look around. Go get some lanterns and meet me at the gate." Brother went off to recruit a few more boys. They searched all around the mouth of the valley for Ramon, but he was nowhere to be seen. They finally gave up. "We'll come back first thing in the morning," said Brother, "We can't do any more tonight. It's too dark." So they trudged back to Kalawao.

The next morning another search party set out. They combed the mouth of the valley but found nothing. "We better go all the way in," said Brother worriedly. They went in and at the foot of the falls, they found Ramon hanging over the basin of water holding on for dear life. He was in a delirious state. They carried Ramon home and put him to bed. After a few days, he became lucid. "Well, you gave us a fright!" said Brother "What happened to you?"

"I don't know, Bruddah," answered Ramon. "I wuz walking along and alla sudden, I see dis beautiful lady wid long blonde hair."

"Go on," said Brother in the voice of authority.

"Well, she stay standin by da road goin to Waihanau. She look at me an make da kine sign foa me to follow," he shrugged. "So I did. When I get close, I can see dis ain't no human, so I get scared an try run back, but no can. Something get the kine grip on me an I no can run. Funny kine dis! Den she made da kine sign to follow in Waihanau. Poho dis kine, I gotta follow. She stay stop at da basin an jumped in. She tell me follow. Bruddah, me scared. I grab da rock wid all my might an hang on. Something try push me in but I hang on. Den she dive down under one rock an by-m-by I see one lizard come out. Den I don't know any more." Ramon recovered and I think the moral of that story is: "NEVER TRUST A BLONDE."

Then Alec, one of our old timers, told me about a cave in Kalawao. As a young boy, Alec lived with an old Hawaiian couple. One night, the old man went to Alec and woke him up. "Eh, ged up. We gotta go somewhere."

"At dis time of night?" protested Alec. As Alec dressed, the old man trimmed a kerosene lamp. Then they set out for Kalawao.

"I have one dream," said the old man. "I wuz tole to go to one cave. When we ged der, we can take anyting we want from da cave. But we gotta watch out. Der are two caves, one next to da odah. Da one wid a skull on spears in front, we no go in. Da odah, okay."

"How we a gonna find one cave in da dark?" grumbled Alec. He wasn't interested in caves and treasures at this time of night.

"Dey tell me foa how find da place." He proceeded to tell Alec how to find it. Sure enough, when they reached the spot, a huge rock rolled back and there was a hole in the ground. Stone steps led down to the cave. As the dream had said, there was a double cave and one was barred by two crossed spears. They did not even look into this cave. The other one was a huge room. One side had niches in which were remains. On the ground was an outrigger canoe with helmets and feather capes. The old man was told that they could take anything they wanted, so Alec tried on a feather helmet but it was too large. He threw it back. Neither of them took anything. When they climbed back out, the stone rolled into place.

This is a very strange place where spirits are reported to roam at will. Hopefully tomorrow I will hear more fascinating history. If I do, I will share it with you in my next letters. God bless you.

With Aloha,

Sr. Wilma

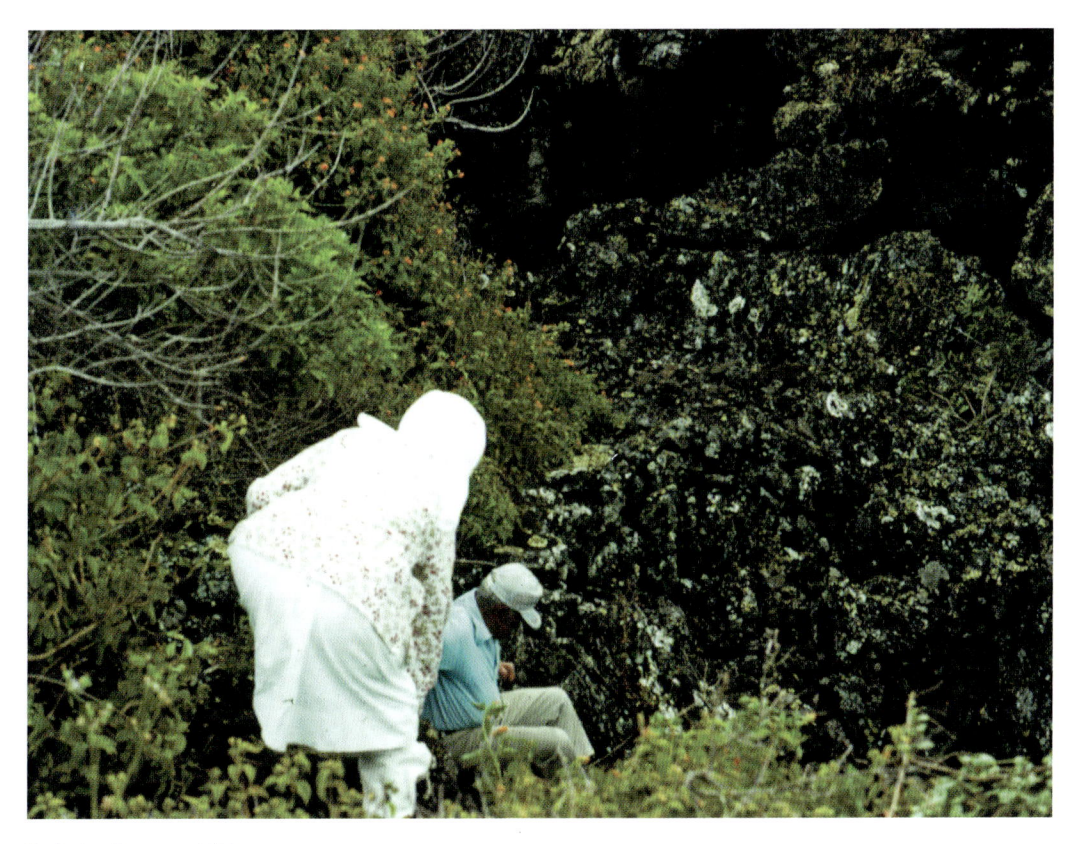

Exploring the caves at Kalaupapa.

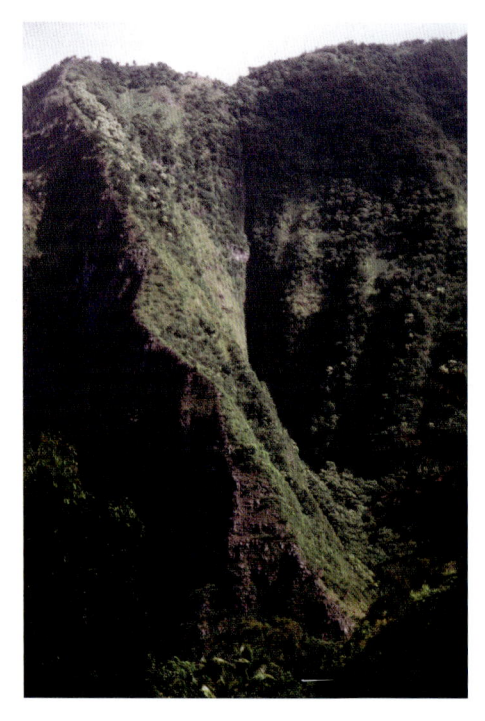

The Mountains leading to Waikolu Valley.

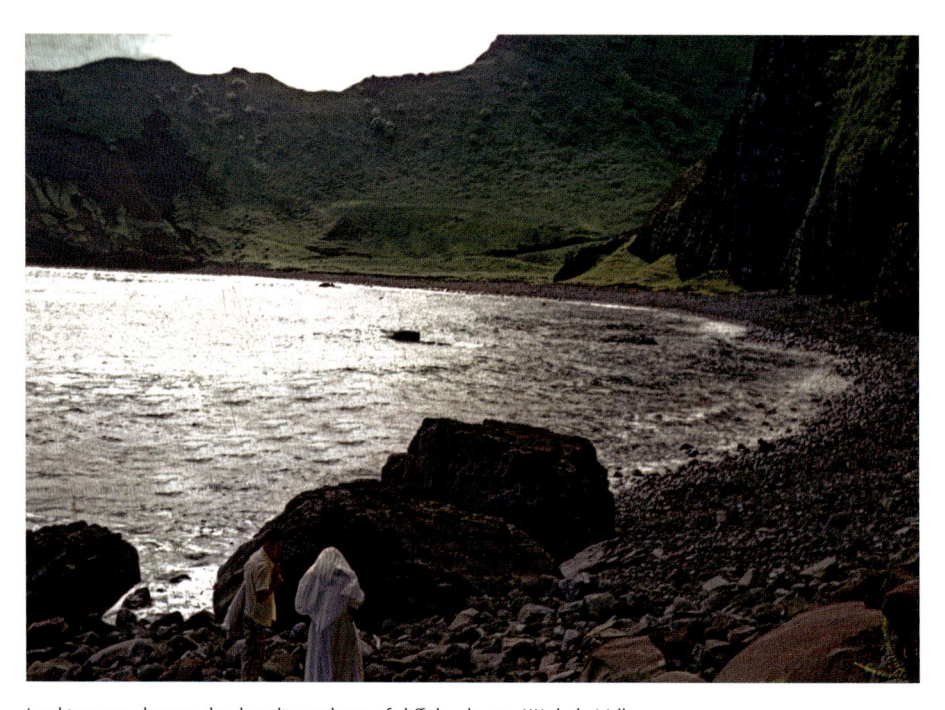

Looking east along rocky shoreline at base of cliffs leading to Waikolu Valley.

Hunting

Dear Sister:

Here I am again with a tale. I hope that you are not getting bored to distraction. Life seems to be full of challenges. This time for me, a mountain, but the old Indian proverb seems to have the answer:

> A small man weighs what can hinder him,
> and fearful, does not set to work.
> Difficulties cause the average man to leave off
> what he has begun.
> A truly great man does not slacken in carrying out
> what he has begun, although obstacles tower
> a thousand-fold until he has succeeded.

About a week or so ago, time flies, the doorbell of the convent rang and I went to answer it. One of our people was leaning over the gate. His jalopy was parked behind him. The inscription on the machine was "Old Black Joe."

"Hey, Sister, you're just the one I want to see," said Ed. I hurried down the steps.

"Good Lord, Ed, what happened to you?" He was all covered with blood, and the seat of his pants was missing.

"Phooey, Hunters!" He spat neatly over the fence. "Me and some guys were hunting wild pigs in Waikolu today. We wuz doing OK when one of those buggers charged us. You know what those guys did?"

"No," I answered spellbound, "What?"

"They took to the trees, that's what, and there wuz me and the dogs all alone. Old Blackie -- he's got more guts than brains -- met the boar head on. Pow!

The old boar just hooked his tusk in Blackie's jaw and threw him about eight feet in the air. I wuz afraid to shoot because there wuz so much dog and boar mixed together. Then King jumped in to help Blackie, and the mean cuss of a boar ripped a hole clean through King's chest. Then he came for me -- he took the seat of my pants -- but I got em, Sister!" He spat neatly over the fence again. "I shoulda had women with me; they woulda been more help."

"You shouldn't be too hard on the guys, Ed. The adrenal glands are funny things, you know. A few weeks ago, we had some visiting Sisters who wanted to see Waialeia Valley so I took them out . . ."

"Wuzn't that kind of stupid? You just had surgery." Our people are outspoken.

"I know, but what can one do? Anyway we were walking along and talking when there was a crashing noise and I was almost eyeball to eyeball with a wild steer. The next thing I knew, I was sitting on the branch of a tree looking down at him. I must have run straight up the tree."

"Yeah," he said dubiously. "Well, what I wanted to ask wuz, could you patch up my dogs? They're in pretty bad shape."

"I'll make a deal with you," I answered. "I promised someone in Hawaii that I'd get a live kid for her little boy. If you take me hunting, I'll patch up your dogs."

"Okay, it's a deal. I'll meet you at the hospital." He jumped into the jalopy and blasted off. Incidentally, we do all kinds of odd nursing at the hospital.

The following week we formed a hunting party. Sister Linus was visiting from Hilo, and I told her that she would have to take the kid back with her.

"You must be out of your mind! I'm not babysitting any goat!"

"Oh yes, you are," I answered sweetly. "Do you want to go hunting with us or not?"

"Sure, I'm game for anything once," she grumbled. So we started off through the jungle: men, dogs, rifles and nuns. The closer we got to the foot of the mountain, the worse it looked, all 2,000 feet of it.

"I don't know how you're going to climb that mountain in those clothes," Ed, the pessimist, said. "+ It gets rougher all the time." We were in a gulch struggling from one huge boulder to another. I was puffing like a steam engine.

"Never mind the clothes; just lead the way!" I answered grimly. I didn't think that my lungs and heart would hold out, but I wouldn't give anyone the satisfaction of knowing it. Sister Linus' face was purple with heat and exertion. I don't know what mine looked like. We managed to struggle half way up the mountain when I stepped on a loose rock, lost my balance, and shot down the mountain side. I splattered on a huge slab of stone jutting out of the cliff. It was an old heiau that I had heard about from the old folks. From the look of the hunters' faces when they reached me, I'm sure that they thought I was dead.

"Don't worry, boys, there's still plenty of steam left in the old girl yet." I stood up shakily. "Let's go."

One of the boys took out a piece of chalk from his pocket and said solemnly, "I'm going to write: 'Sister splashed down here.'"

After the slab was duly blessed, we began to climb again. Suddenly the dogs made a silent dash and the boys disappeared after them just as silently. There was a shot and the bleating of goats. When Sister and I arrived, the dogs had a beautiful tiny kid encircled.

The shot had frightened off the herd, but the little one was too slow. The boys carried him down the mountain, bleating and kicking all the way. We took him to the convent and had to bottle feed him because he was only a few days old with the umbilical cord still hanging. A few days later, he went to Hawaii with Sister. Later I received a letter from Sister saying that she didn't have to baby-sit. The kid made such a hit with the passengers that some of them offered to baby-sit him. Little Tommy was thrilled with his pet and Mrs. Smith was tearing her hair because the goat was eating everything in sight — especially her prized plants. Well, you can't have everything! Will write to you later. In the meantime, walk with God.

            With Aloha,

            Sr. Wilma

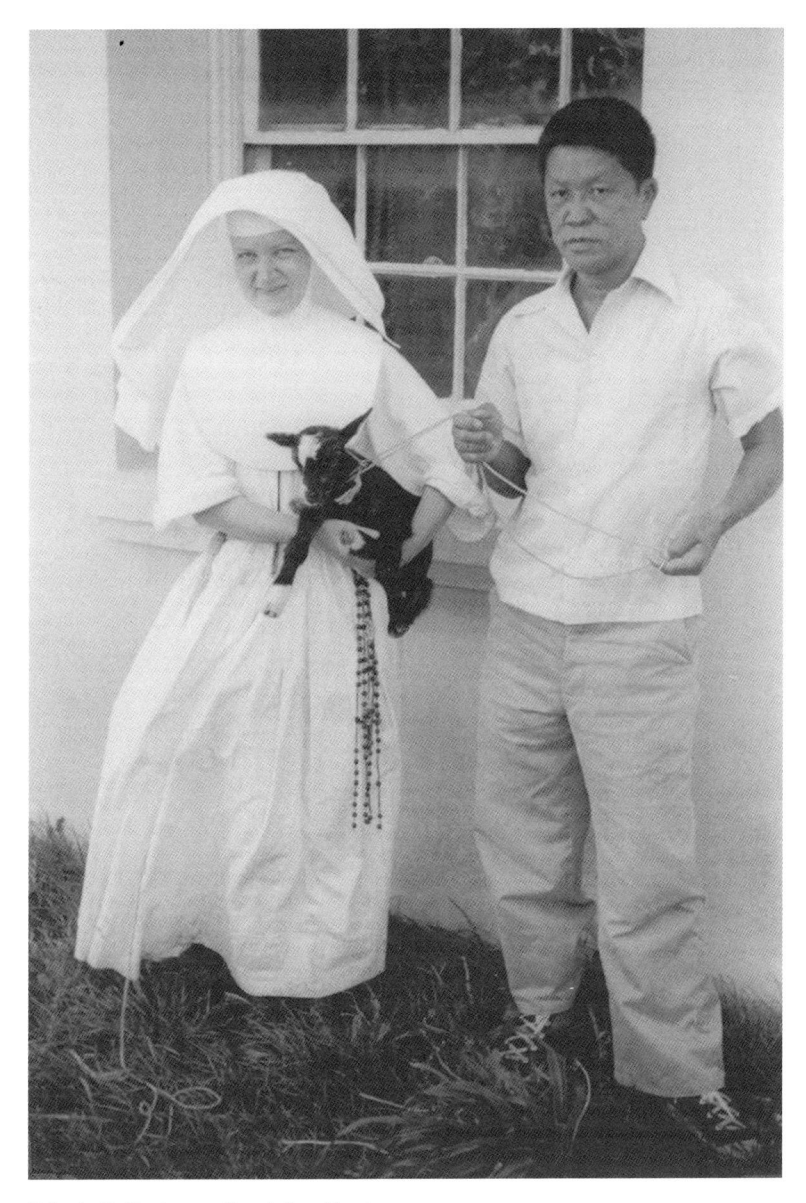

"Billy the Kid" taken to Church for a Blessing.

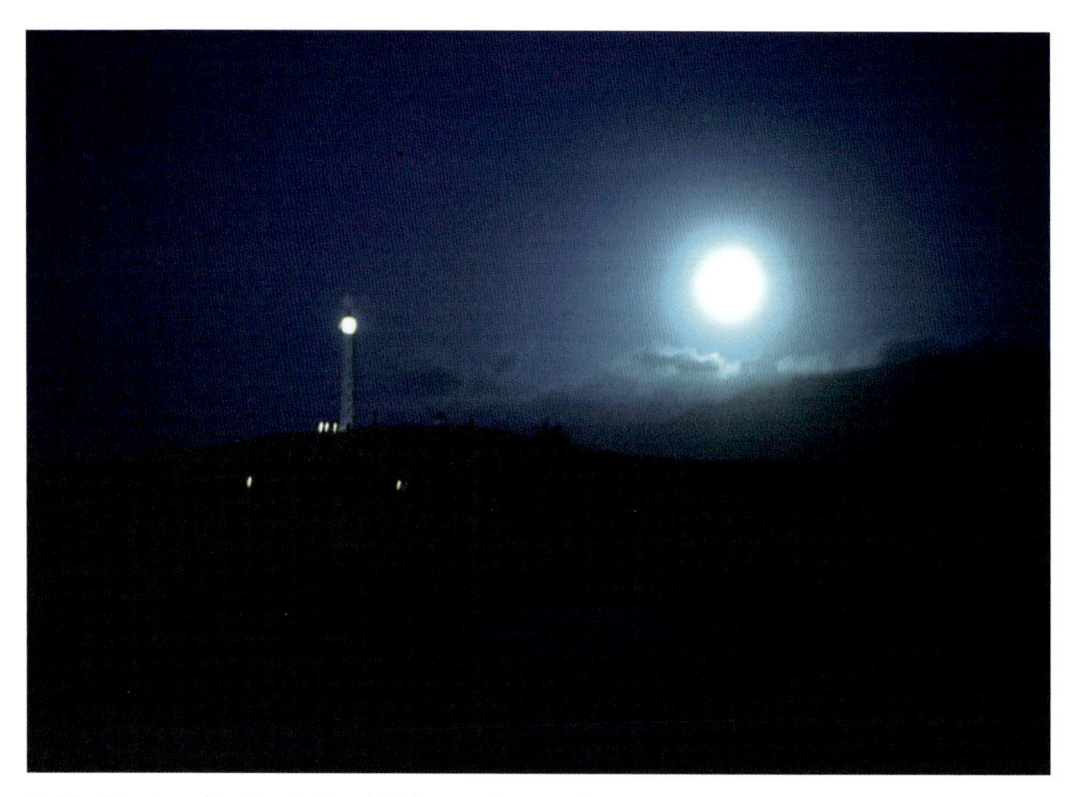

Molokai, "Daughter of the Moonlight", with lighthouse in foreground

Night Duty

Dear Sister,

Well, it's that time again. I'm on night duty. I truly hate that shift, first because it seems that the spirits of the Settlement come to romp, and second, the work is heavy. Thank God that when we have one of our parishioners critical, our holy pastor Father Peter stays with them all night so that I'm not alone. Our people speak very matter of factly about death. I remember one of our patients had a lovely white dress made for Easter. Everyone told her how lovely it was so she said to me, "Sister, I changed my mind. I'm not going to wear this for Easter. I'll save it for my funeral."

I laughed. "Why, Frances, you aren't going to die for years!"

"I hope you will be here when I die, Sister. I want you to dress me. Now, if you could buy for me a blue velvet ribbon about two inches wide and long enough to make a bow, I'll use that for a belt."

"For heaven's sake, what makes you think that you are going to die?" I asked.

"Never mind. When you dress me, tie the ribbon in front. Turn me a little bit on my left side in the coffin and put the picture of my dear husband in my right arm. And don't let that Louisa visit my coffin or I'LL HAUNT HER! She caused me enough trouble in life."

A few months later, Frances accidentally fell out of bed while turning on her side. I took x-rays but the doctor could not find anything wrong. The next morning as I came on duty, the orderly met me at the door. "Sister, Frances wants to see you right away." I hurried to her room.

"Sister, I want to be anointed."

"Now, Frances?" I asked surprised.

"Yes, right away."

The pastor came quickly and anointed her. A half hour later the nurse was bathing her. She appeared at my door out of breath. "Sister, I think Frances is dying!" By the time we arrived at her room, Frances was gone. It was a shock to everyone. So I dressed her in her white dress with the blue ribbon but I took a chance on Louisa. I didn't tell her not to visit the coffin. As far as I know, Frances didn't come back to haunt her. I'm sure she had much better things to do on the other side.

Another time one of my favorite patients, a cardiac patient, was sitting up in bed crocheting when I went in to visit her. "What a lovely piece, Mary," I exclaimed. She was pleased.

"Do you like it, Sister?"

"Oh, yes. I think it's exquisite."

Mary's condition became progressively worse. One day I went in to check on her and found her sitting up in bed crocheting. Her color was bad and her breathing labored. I said, "Mary, you should not be exerting yourself like that. You had better put that away and rest."

"But, Sister, I want to finish this for you before I die." What can one say to that?

At Kalaupapa we don't embalm our dead. The nurse prepares the body and he or she is buried the same day unless the death has occurred late in the day, or if a relative has to fly in for the funeral. The services are tranquil and somehow intimate. The body is taken to the respective parish hall and lies in state until the services in church begin. The hall is banked with our beautiful Hawaiian flowers. In the Catholic hall, the body is flanked by a large crucifix and candles. The Settlement turns out for each funeral.

In our hall, the pastor preceeded by two acolytes carrying the ceremonial crucifix, incense, and holy water enters and begins the prayers. Our pastor then blesses the body. After that, we file past the coffin and bid "Aloha" to our friend. We then go in procession behind the coffin into the church for services. After Mass, Father again blesses and incenses the coffin while saying, "Go forth, Christian soul. May the angels lead you to paradise . . ." As the coffin is wheeled out, the choir sings:

> O Paradise, O Paradise, who would not seek for rest?
> Who would not seek the happy land,
> where they that love are blessed?

We follow the ambulance to the cemetery. The coffin is laid next to the excavated earth which will shortly receive it. We gather around the grave site and say prayers in unison. The soft soughing of the wind in the ironwood trees and the soft murmur of the sea can be heard as we pray. The coffin is lowered and covered with earth. We wait until this is finished and the mound is covered with flowers. Our brother or sister traverses the great highway of death and we return to walk the difficult path of the living.

One night I was very busy and the orderlies said, "Sister, why don't you eat your supper and we'll stay up to answer bells; otherwise you won't eat." I gratefully accepted and in my hurry, I spilled some milk.

"Never mind, Sister, eat," said Mariah, "I'll get the mop and wipe it up." She ran out to get the mop which was hanging on the rail of the ramp leading to the women's ward. She was back in breakneck speed, looking ashen. I dropped my sandwich, frightened.

"What happened, Mariah?"

"Sister, I was just almost killed!" she panted.

"For heaven's sake, how?"

"I was going to pick up the mop, and this HUGE rock shrieked past my head!" she wailed.

"Keep calm, Mariah. You know that's nonsense. It's impossible for a rock to hurl past that ramp unless it's shot from a cannon suspended in the sky. I'll get the mop."

I ran down the hall with Mariah wailing like a banshee. "You'll be killed, you'll be killed!"

I yanked the door open and stooped over to get the mop. This probably saved my life because, as I bent over, a huge rock zoomed past my head like a guided missile. I was so angry that I ran down the ramp and flashed my light over the roof, in the palm trees and under the hospital. The hospital is built on stilts. Meanwhile Mariah kept yelling, "Come back in; you'll be killed." I took her advice and dashed back in and slammed the door shut. I wiped the milk up with paper towels. To this day, I have no idea who hurled that rock at me.

Still another night around one o'clock, I was sitting at the desk with my feet twined around the rungs of the chair when the most spine-chilling scream split the air. I jumped up and promptly fell to the floor with my feet still entwined. The screams continued from one of the women's wards. As I dashed down the hall, I wondered why all the call bells were not ringing in alarm. When I reached the ward, the screaming stopped. I was so unnerved; I had to lean against the door for a few seconds. Then I ran to each bed to see who had been murdered. All but one in the ward were peacefully sleeping. I went over to the sleepless patient and asked, "Taki, how long have you been awake?"

"Quite a long time, Sister. Why?"

"Who screamed in the ward just now?"

"No one, Sister."

"Are you sure, Taki?"

"Yes, Sister. I'm positive." I didn't want to press her further on the subject.

"Do you want anything for sleep?"

"No, Sister. I'm all right." I could hardly walk back to the desk, I was so shaken up. I don't know who screamed, but whoever it was, seemed in mortal agony. Or perhaps I had just dozed off after a hard day at work.

What a place this is! Perhaps when you come to visit, you'll see one of our famous fire balls which whiz through the air seeking its target. The idea is to keep out of its way. A disgruntled member of our parish sent one after our Father Peter. He dashed into the church and slammed the door before it got him, thank God.

If I survive this round of nights, I'll write again. Keep well and may God keep you in the palm of His hand.

                                              With Aloha,

                                              Sr. Wilma

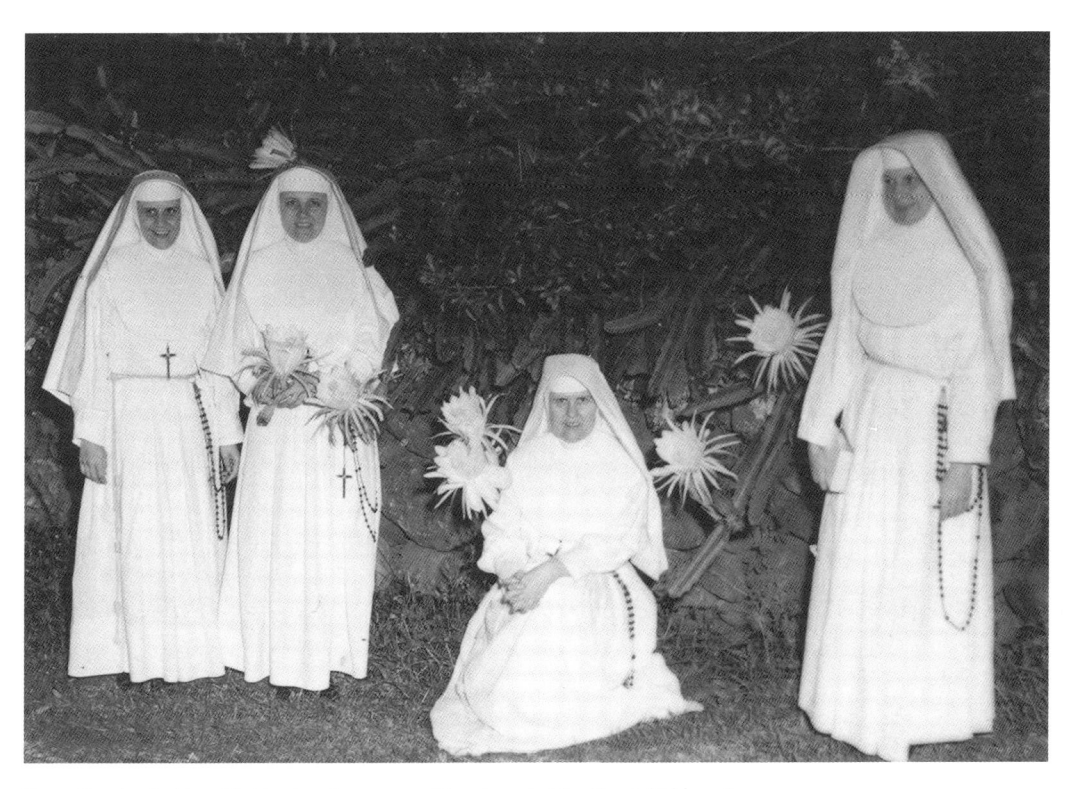

Sisters Gaudentia, Mary Christopher, Rosanne and Francine admiring the night-blooming cereus.

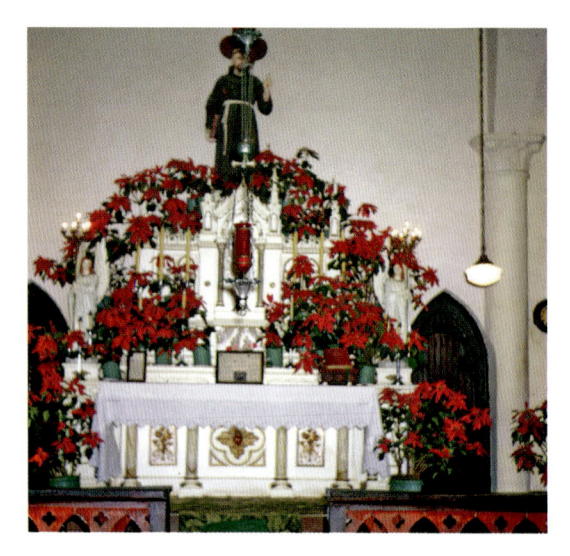

The high altar at St. Francis Church with poinsettias.

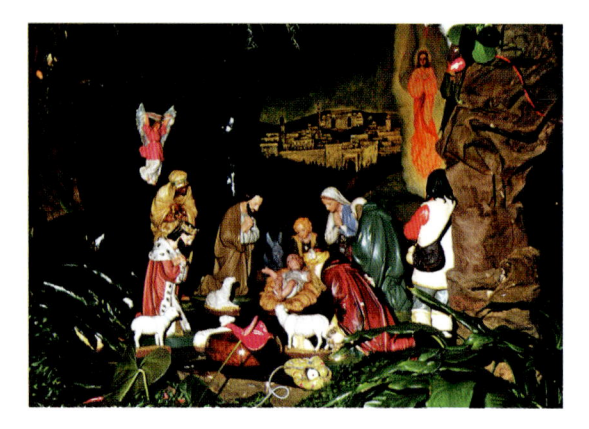

The crib.

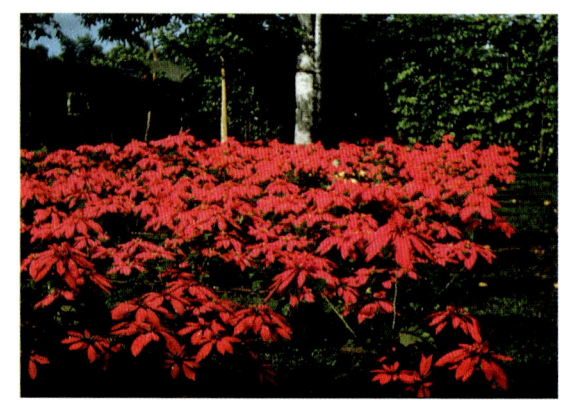

Poinsettias blooming in the Protestant church yard.

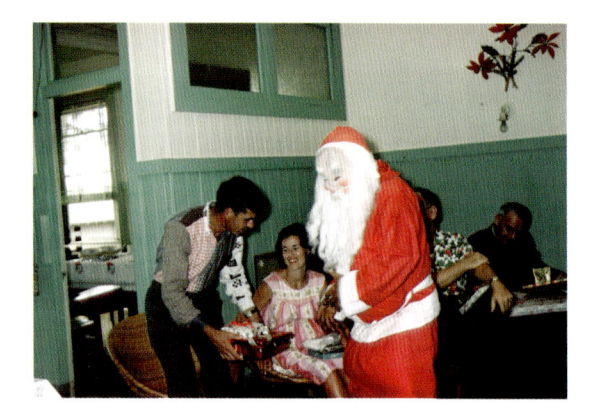

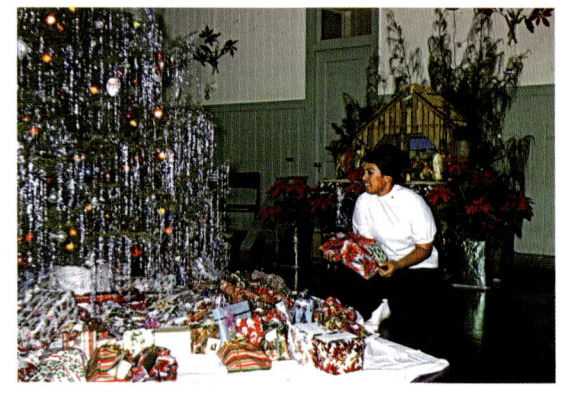

Santa Claus visits the hospital.

Kuulei Bell helping Santa

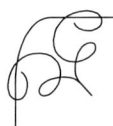

Christmas – Kalaupapa Style

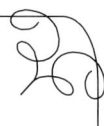

Dear Sister,

It is difficult to realize that Christmas is only a few weeks away, especially since there isn't any snow on the ground. I thought that you may be interested in hearing how they tell the story of Christmas in the islands. I think the following was put together by Dr. Nathaniel B. Emerson.

Da Very First Christmas

Once upon a times . . . . Long ago and far away – wuz one man name Lokepa, an his wife wuz called Mele. It just so happen around dat times da king tink he like get one list of all da folks who stay live inside da country, so he send out da word dat errybody betta go sign up wid da mayor in his home town.

About da same times, da Angel tell Mele she going get one Keiki…

But Lokepa, he put Mele on top his Kona Nightengale – dat's Hawaiian kine donkey, you know, an dey go holoholo his town wich wuz call Betlehema.

When dey get ovah dat place, so many folks wuz der awready, get no place foa stop excep inside one barn, an dat wuz where Lokepa an Mele stay.

On dat night, one leedle boy wuz born…Mele wrap him up all nice an warm an make one leedle bed on top da straw — an she pick out one nice name foa da keiki.

She call him IESU.

Now in da meantimes, wuz tree wise ole men who been read an study foa long times. Biemby, dey find out dat pretty soon one keiki going be born who going be king. Dey tink so day like find dis keiki, show der aloha!

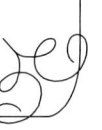

So dey get all dressed up in fancy clothes trim wid gold an silver on top, an each one carry da kine presants foa give da keiki. Den dey can see one big star inside da sky, so dey go ovah dat place. Biemby dey come to one town so dey stop, try find out if dat's where da keiki get born who going be king.

When da king hear dis, he get planty worried an huhu! "Gee," he tink himself, "if dis keiki really going be king, den someday I going be poho!" So he call his kahunas togedda an he say, "Eh, what dis kine? Errybody say one keiki get born who going be king!" An da kahunas dey tell him, "Yehyehyehyeh, dat's right! You know why? Caz da kahu he say dis keiki going get born inside da leedle town of Bethlehema!"

So da king invite da tree wise ole men come see em, an he make da kine Hoomalimali, tell em dey real smath an all like dat. Den he say, "When you find em, lemme know, yeh? Cuz I like see em too!" But all dis times he really want make sure da keiki get put outa da way, so he can nevah be king!!

[Boy, crooked like one hau tree, dis guy!] So da tree wise ole men, dey come to Bethlehem dy find Lokepa an Mele an da leedle Iesu. An dey kneel down in front of da keiki, an dey open up all dose prasents: gold, an da most rare perfumes dey can find…

Dat night when da tree wise ole men wuz sleeping, get one dream: It tell em, more betta dey go right home — no need go back see da king. So next day, dey pack up an go home anadah way – so dat king, he nevah get his hands on da keiki!

So dat leedle Iesu he grow up wise an strong, an he teach folks da best way foa live is try get aloha foa your neighbor, an try da same ting foa da odda guy dat you like em do foa you.

Pretty soon, folks stath call Iesu "Christ" [which mean alla same ting, Savior"] an so dat's how his birthday get to be called "Christmas."

****

I was interrupted in writing this letter so it is now January the seventh. The three wise men have come and gone. The Christmas season is over — how quickly it passes. Here on Molokai it is still Christ's birthday. Several months before Christmas on a clear evening, the church choirs can be heard practicing their music. The drama department also begins early to prepare its contribution. This year it will be "Ahmal and the Night Visitors." There are mysterious trips to the craft shop. Everyone who is able, strings outdoor lights around his home. When the sun sinks in the west, which is incidentally called "He ala nei a ka maki" or "The great highway of death," all the lights go on in the Settlement and it becomes a shimmering fairyland.

Several days before Christmas, a crew of volunteers armed with hammers, nails, boards, and canvas filched from the hospital, build the large, beautiful crib which adorns our Catholic Church. The church is scrubbed by loving hands and the whole church is filled with huge poinsettia plants which have been carefully tended by a patient who is almost completely blind. The church really looks fit for the newborn King!

Then at midnight, when all things are in silence, the church bells ring and our solemn high Mass begins. At the consecration, the gossamer veil between the celestial realms and earth are parted, and again the Almighty Word comes down from heaven to take on our mortal flesh and teach us how to live. But how few listen!

Everyone who is able to stand on his feet is in church to greet the newborn King. After Mass as the organ peals "Joy to the World" the congregation files up to the crib, the more fortunate ones leading the blind and the lame, to place their offering in the calabash which is placed there. The Sisters and some of the congregation stay on for the celebration of the Mass at dawn. I just love that Mass at dawn. It is very special to me.

Now that the holy season is over, the decorations in the Settlement have been taken down, and it somehow looks very empty. The convent decorations came down last night. Sisters Marie and Claudia had just walked up to the attic with the last load and had packed it away under the critical eyes of "Happy," our dog, when Sister Marie said, "Well, that's all. Goodbye." The next moment there was a tremendous crash. Startled, Sister Claudia spun around. Happy was looking down incredulously through a gaping hole in the attic floor which is directly over our community room. In the community room we have a long table around which we sit at recreation.

Sister Claudia dashed down the stairs yelling, "Help!" This brought the rest of us running. On the table, stretched out in a faint was Sister Marie with a basket of flowers on her chest. The flowers had flown off the table when Sister landed. For a moment we thought that Sister was dead. The superior immediately called the doctor who gave Sister expert care. After the excitement died down, we all trooped back into the community room to assess the damage. After a moment of contemplation, our superior said, "We just can't tell the administrator that someone walked through the ceiling; we'll have to put up a new ceiling tonight."

"Where are we going to find material to fix it with?" someone asked.

Sister Claudia, always the practical one, said, "There is a piece just the right size in the cottage which they are tearing down."

So several of the stronger Sisters dragged the kanek [pressed board] to the convent and with a great deal of perspiration and muscle strain, we put up the new ceiling. It took us until past midnight to finish the job. We could go into the carpentry business if things get rough by the looks of the ceiling. We are now valiantly carrying on while Sister Marie lies in bed, black and blue all over and stiff as a board. Take a lesson, dear, and stay away from shaky attic floors.

May your New Year be filled with God's blessings.

With Aloha,

Sr. Wilma

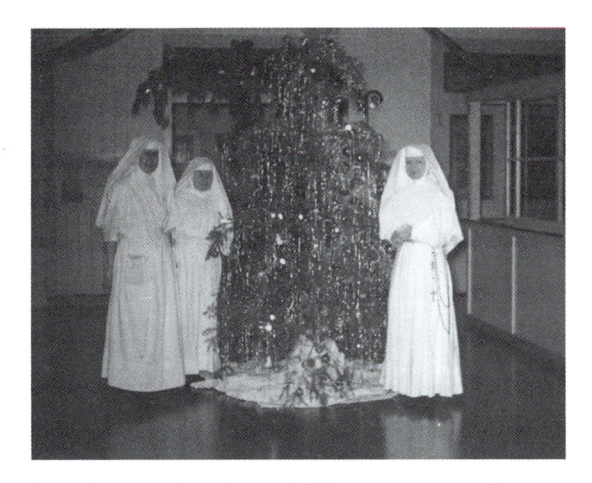

Sisters Rosanne, Carmelita and Wilma trimming the Christmas tree at the hospital.

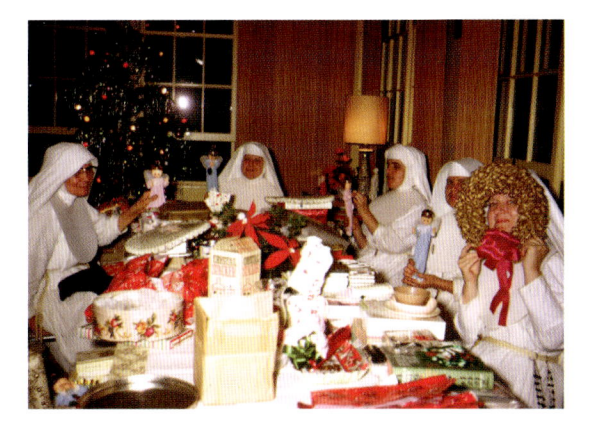

Sisters opening Christmas gifts at the Bishop Home Convent.

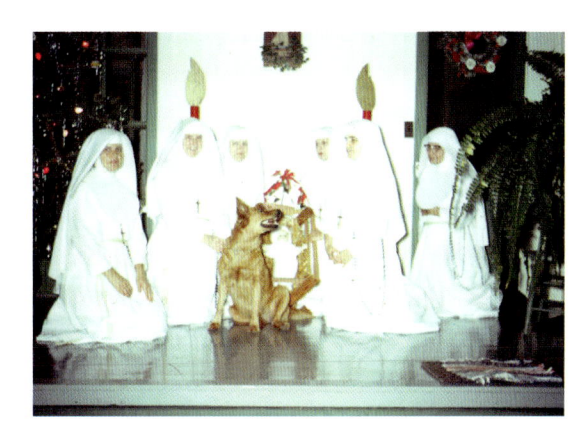

Sisters with "Happy" at Christmas.

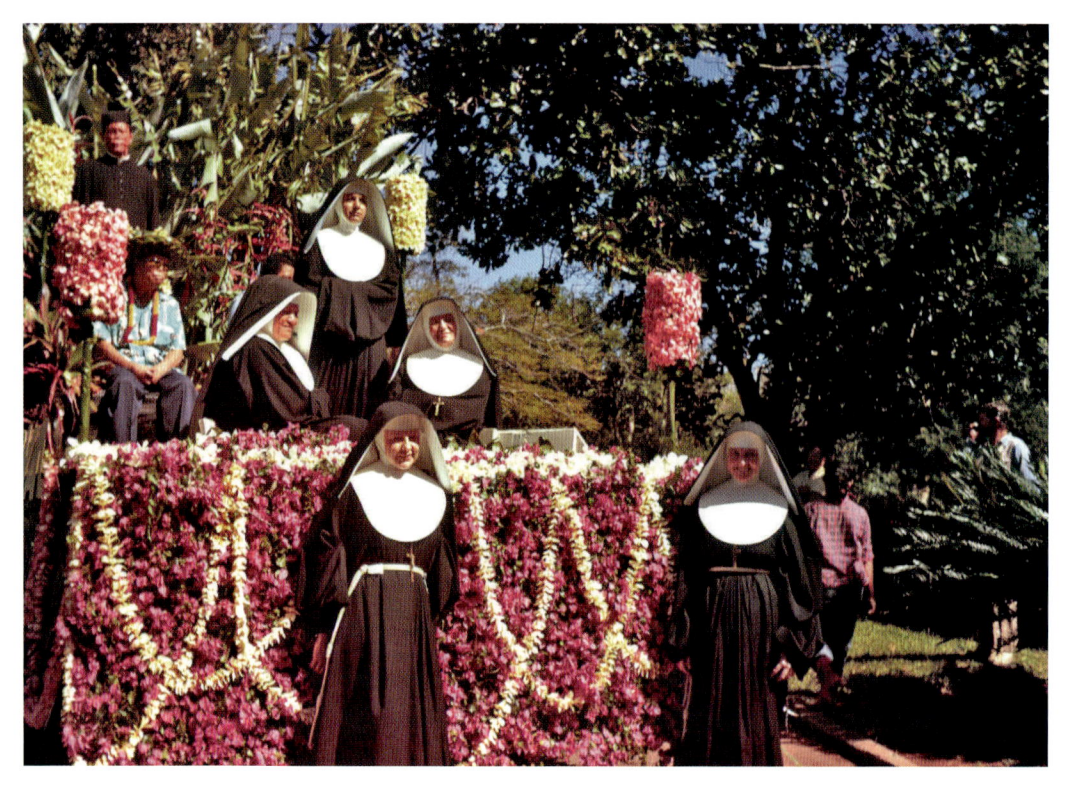

The sulfones gave people a new lease on life. This float with residents dressed in sisters' habits, was part of a parade marking the anniversary of Mother Marianne's death.

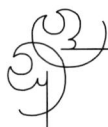

New Treatment

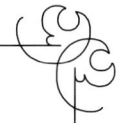

July, 1946

Dear Sister,

Hopefully, this is the dawn of a new era. Last night our medical director called us all together, patients and workers, to outline our new program for treatment of Hansen's Disease. I know you will be interested in reading it!

"I have called you here tonight because we are about to expand our treatment program, and I want to explain to you who are interested what we have in mind, what we are about to do, and what we hope to do, and give you a clear idea of where we stand.

"We now hope to give active special treatment to every patient who wants it, whose physical condition justifies it, and who will give full cooperation as described below. Now, the question is, what do we mean by active treatment? Some people get the idea that because we have not given Chaulmoogra oil during the past year since our predecessor, with whom I agree, decided that it did not accomplish anything, that Kalaupapa is nothing but a hotel. This is not born out by statistics. Our records show that as a result of hospitalization, careful nursing care, use of drugs such as the sulfonamides and penicillin, transfusions, etc., we have been able to accomplish something. During the life of Father Damien, the average length of life here was three and one half years. When Father Peter came, the average length of life was eight years, our statistics for those dying the last years show the average length of life to be eighteen years. Certainly we know there are comparatively fewer dressings compared to previously, probably largely because of new drugs which we have used locally for the ulcers.

"But to many people the word treatment means something special—in the days of chaulmoogra oil, it was chaulmoogra oil – in the days of Diphtheria toxoid, it was Diphtheria toxoid – whether it was good or not, that was the treatment, and nothing else counted. Today it is Promin. A lot of you have been reading the "*Star.*" I read it too. The patients at Carville are over enthusiastic – they talk as if it were a cure-all. I wish that were true. No doctor claims that Promin cures leprosy. Of those treated, only a small percentage becomes negative and are paroled.

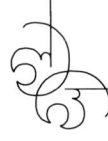

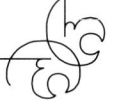

"On our present schedule we give seven patients five grams of Promin six days a week for three months and then a week's rest. We may change that schedule. We have to start slowly and expand slowly. The present patients have been on treatment for four months, but it is still too soon to tell the results.

"The thing I want to make plain right now is that I hope your hopes will not be raised too high. Probably many of you will be helped, but Promin is not a cure – some patients may not improve, some may get worse; most patients improve. In one recent publication that came out of Carville, they had a pretty picture of a pair of legs with ulcers before Promin and after two years of treatment with Promin showing most of the ulcers healed. I didn't think this was even a particularly good ad. We have been able to do the same thing here just using local treatment of ulcers without Promin.

Mr. Stein, who visited Carville recently said that the thing that struck him most was the scarcity of dressings. But we must still remember that Carville started using Promin four years ago at about the same time we started using sulfonamides, that we have been able to accomplish locally a lot with sulfa drugs and that where the results on Promin as published by Carville may look very good, they may not seem as dramatic here because we have already made so much progress in the same direction.

"A good many of the patients who have started on the drug have not been able to continue it. Of the first sixty-six started on Diazole at Carville, thirty-one stopped. It would not be so bad now that we have learned what to do for some of the toxic reactions. Of the first sixty-eight on Promin, sixteen were unable to continue the treatment, but for those who can take it, this is what it may do:

1. Nodules and infiltrations shrink.

2. Ulcers heal (while it is stated that ulcers tend to heal, nothing is said about those ulcers that are associated with bad bone, i.e. toes and fingers).

3. Noses improved.

4. Mouth and throat lesions improve. At the present time there are only two patients wearing tubes at Carville, but don't blame this on Promin

as they do not have so severe a grade of leprosy there, as we have here. They have never had the number of tubes there as we have here, but they do feel that Promin has helped to reduce the number of tubes.

5. Eye lesions become stationary and sometimes improve. They are not, by any means, all improved by Promin, but what it seems to do is to stop the eye from getting worse, and, in a few cases, there is actual improvement in vision.

6. Only one report is available on a nerve case. This one showed slight improvement.

7. Of ten T.B. cases treated, two got worse, and eight improved. Of course, this could have happened without Promin. When improvement occurs, it is slow and we do not expect to see any definite improvement before six months or longer. Because of this, we ask every person who takes the treatment of promin, that if his condition warrants and the doctors think he should, he will continue treatment for a year."

As yet, the only drug we have on hand is Promin. You will remember that I spoke to you about two others which have been promised to us to try out – one is yet without a name, and the other, Pyricidin. I hope there will not be too much of a rush for Promin as yet, as one of these other drugs may be better. In considering the various drugs, until there has been further trial, we can not say which one is best, and we would like to try all available drugs until this can be determined.

<u>General Considerations</u>
To start treatment with any of the Promin series, you need:

1. Good veins for those given by vein (Promin and Diptoside).

2. Fairly good blood. A patient with a red count below 2,300,000 will not be started on treatment. We will attempt to build up his blood first.

3. Fairly good kidneys.

4. Fairly good liver. If we ever agree to give this drug to a patient with a bad liver and/or kidneys, it will be definitely at his own risk.

Before starting treatment on anyone, we will want a complete physical and laboratory examination, and as many photos as we can take. Pictures will be for our records and none will be published without the consent of the patient. Patients will be required to have blood counts and urinalysis at frequent intervals.

I bring up the subject of dressings because I think that any person taking one of the drugs should let us watch his sores and help in taking care of them. If you are taking a treatment and you do not feel well in any way, we expect you to report immediately.

I feel that anyone whose veins are poor and any of the younger children should wait until we can get the drugs that can be taken by mouth. I would like some of those whose leprosy is not too active to wait until some of the newer drugs are available.

Present Program in Summary

1. Present Promin here and from Kalihi to continue.

2. Quinacrine patients to continue.

3. Children and poor vein patients to wait for drugs which can be given by mouth.

4. Hold relatively inactive patients for newer drugs.

5. Start Promin in a few weeks on active cases, especially those having poor eyes, many chronic ulcers, poor throats, and frequent reactions.

So we embark on a new venture and everyone is hoping that this is the answer which we have been looking for since antiquity. The newspapers give a conservative view of the new program, but we on Molokai carry the torch of hope.

This is an elusive disease indeed. The clinical picture can vary with locality and presents many unsolved problems. For thousands of years, it has carried a social stigma which is unjustifiable. It would be well for all to keep in mind a

Gospel story which aptly describes the idea of stigma. "Who sinned, this man or his parents?" The question is asked by the righteous Pharisees, their phylacteries rustling importantly, as with bated breath they await the verdict of Christ.

"Neither this man nor his parents," answered Christ. What a letdown for the scandal mongers!

In the name of progress we have changed the name of leprosy to Hansen's Disease. It is a sin of great magnitude to call it by name. It is only logical that if we wish to educate the public, we should begin by teaching that leprosy is not a dirty word but a disease like the thousands of diseases which plague the world. Also, leprosy is much less contagious than many other diseases. Fortunately, the families of most of the patients suffering the disease accept the fact. This however is not true of all families. Two letters from our files illustrate the different attitudes:

Memo:

To: Supt, Bd of Hospitals and Settlement
From: Resident Physician
Subject: Relative of ___(name withheld)_____

Have you any information regarding _____'s relatives and their present address? He has particularly mentioned his daughter from whom he would like to hear. He is old and his general condition very poor, and even a little gesture as a letter from her would mean a good deal to him. Will you please see what you can do?

                            _____
                            Resident Physician
                            Kalaupapa

The daughter had no time for the broken old man who only asked for a letter. He died without hearing from the family. Then there is the letter which restores our faith in mankind again.

Hilo, Hawaii
Sept. 29, 1944

Dr. _____, Nurses and Employees of Kalaupapa Pali Station

Dear Friends:

We the parents of the late _____ wish to take this means to express our sincere thanks and appreciation for the splendid care given him during his hospitalization.

We are indeed grateful for all the loving care and friendship shown him, thus making his stay there a very pleasant one until his last moments.

We thank you from the bottom of our hearts in carrying out his last wish by cremating his body and sending his ashes home. It took some time but thanks to you it arrived in perfect condition.

May the Lord help and guide you all in carrying out this wonderful work, helping mankind, who are at your mercy, so that, they may be able to face a brighter future.

Sincerely yours,

_____(Name Withheld_____

In the earliest days of the disease, little was known about the treatment of it. The Board of Health felt that segregation would take care of the problem. At the settlement only the simplest of medications were kept, namely soothing ointments for the ulcers and purgatives. They felt that purgatives would cure all ills. The patients planted eucalyptus trees to use as steam inhalation, tea, and steam baths. One of the old timers from the 1800s stated positively that the steam bath helped a great deal even causing nodules to disappear.

The government sent Dr. Hillibrand to Japan to learn what he could about the treatment of leprosy. In 1886, the treatment of Dr. Goto began to be used and seemed to be of some benefit to the patients at Kakaako, the receiving station on Oahu. Father Damien took the treatment for a while but finally gave it up as a lost cause. Dr. Mouritz tells us about it in his book, The Path of the Destroyer:

> "Early in the year 1887 Fr. Damien was able to get the much talked of Goto's bathing and medicine established at Kalawao. He proceeded to demonstrate his belief in the treatment by excessive use of both medicines and bathing, using hot water at a temperature of 108* and remaining in the same for hours, drinking tea of the nature of a semi-bitter tonic. Aesculus Turbinate, is part of the treatment, and also a handful of herbs is used in the bath, supposed to dissolve in the water and liberate medicinal properties. Together with all this, a teaspoonful of pills weighing about 2 grams each, was also partaken of daily. After a few weeks of vigorous use of this Goto treatment, it had the effect of giving Fr. Damien a semi-asphyxiated appearance, symptoms of aphonic and dipponia showed up; he tottered in his walk, his clothes appeared like bags hung on his figure, the lobes of his ears became enormously enlarged, almost reaching his collar. Bronchial catarrh, edema of the feet completed the grave symptoms. Yet, in the treatment of his case, he claimed it was doing him good, and he felt better than he had been for the past two years. He lost at least thirty-five pounds in bodily weight at this time…."

The treatment fell from favor but apparently was revived in 1893. The following is from the Hawaiian Star, April 13, 1903.

> Dr. Masanao Goto, the eminent Japanese leprosy specialist, is preparing to make another visit to the . . . . settlement on the island of Molokai. The Doctor will leave Monday for a month's stay together with Mr. David Dayton representing the government Board of Health.
>
> Dr. Goto who has been secured by the Hawaiian government to treat the lepers under restraint has made a life's study of the disease and its treatment as his father S. Goto had before him and professes to have an infallible remedy, a portion of ingredients of his medicine being secret . . . . As to

the doctor's treatment of leprosy, it looks very simple. He uses four kinds of medicine, demanding of the patient only abstinence from liquors, and insisting on the plentiful use of good nutritious food.

The medicine used is made from the oil of the Tai Fuchsia seed, procured in China, and the bark of the Hichigo, a Japanese shrub tree in connection with certain mineral and vegetable salts, the nature of which is kept secret. The internal medicines are given in the form of pellets while the same ingredients in different proportions are added to a sulpherated bath and are used for outward application, the patient being required to bathe freely three times each day with this wash, to take the pellets at certain intervals, and to rub the stiffened joints freely after bathing. This is the entire formula . . . . He says, "The internal remedies persistently combat the germs until they are destroyed while the bath cleanses and heals, and the good food produces new blood and strength which is health . . .

Arrangements will be made to conduct some important scientific investigations . . . . Among the most important experimental studies will be the planting of the bacilli of a [patient] into poi and other food in the effort to discover if the disease may be then transmitted to others. It is the doctor's theory that food is the most common as well as the most potent factor in the communication of leprosy . . . . Doctor Goto believes . . . . that the most subtle infection comes from kissing, as the germs of leprosy invariably infect the nose and the mouth through the mucous membranes . . . . A study of the secretions of [patients] will be made and comparisons with the same from healthy patients will be noted . . . . Doctor Goto has been secured by the Hawaiian government to take charge of the medical department of the [settlement] for the coming year, and in that time the doctor proposes to work some wonderful effects, and, to use his own words, "show the world that leprosy can be effectively cured."

The Inspection of [Patients]

May 11, 1893

. . . The bath being ready on the twenty-fifth, Doctor Goto commenced treating twenty-five persons at the Bishop Home. Sometimes there is sufficient hot water for the bath, other times when there is no force of water in the pipes, there is not a supply of hot water for the bath. It will require a coil to assist the heater from the range in order to do the work well at the Bishop Home, more particularly for the afternoon bath so as to use the same water that was used in the morning.

. . . On the fourth instant, there were ninety-two persons at the boys home and eighty-eight at the Bishop Home and Sister Marianne informed me that there were as many at the homes as there were accommodations for. ...

--- Report by D. Dayton

Sister Leopoldina was in charge of the treatment at Bishop Home. The baths were given from 8:00 a.m. to 11:00 a.m. and from 1:00 p.m. to 2:00 p.m. in two long, high wooden bath tubs which were lined with coils to keep the water hot. Each tub accommodated twelve patients who were required to stand neck deep in the medicated water for twenty minutes. After this, they were taken out and wrapped in blankets. Patients were cooled off gradually. One of our old timers who took the treatment told me that Sister had to be very vigilant because the patients sometimes fainted from the heat and had to be taken out promptly. Strangely enough, the patients stated that no one was ever burned by this water, and that some patients were released as arrested cases after taking the treatment.

The next specific used was chaulmoogra oil. The drug had been used in ancient China and India but was not put into use in the Hawaiian Islands until the late 1800s and that experimentally. It began to be used as a specific in the early 1900s. Not all patients were helped by the medication although some did benefit from it and from its derivatives, the Ethyl Eaters. The drug was taken both by mouth and by injection which, the patients stated, was very painful.

Radium had been used in Paris before 1910 by Dr. Baurmann who felt that it should be used as a symptomatic remedy and would prove to be very beneficial in the future treatment of leprosy. It was used in the Hawaian Islands by Dr. Sandidge between the years 1925-26 as treatment for nasal complications in the disease. He found that it destroyed the lymphoma of the cavity, but not the bacilli which is found in the nose. It also perforated the nasal system and caused its collapse, therefore its use was discontinued. An auxiliary treatment used on Molokai was the "snow stick" or carbonic snow. This was used to burn down the nodules in the lepromatous type. According to the patients who took the treatment, the application of the snow caused ulceration and scarring. It was discontinued as being unbeneficial.

It had been noticed that foreign proteins when used in the treatment of leprosy gave rise to acute lepromatous reactions with high fever, and that after the patient had weathered the storm of reaction, he or she was often much better, the lesions clearing up in many cases, and some patients did not have another flair up for a long time, even for years. It was thought that perhaps the fever was the causative factor in the improvement. So artificial fever was experimented with. At Kalaupapa, it was done with the "sweat box," a home-made imitation of the Kettering hyperthern. The patient was wrapped in blankets and placed in a long wooden box which generated its heat from a series of light bulbs placed in the box. The patient's temperature was elevated to 105° or higher if tolerated. Supportive treatment of fluids and medications was given The patient took a series of these treatments if there were no contraindications, but on the whole the treatment was not well tolerated. So it was discontinued.

In the beginning of the 40's, diphtheria toxoid was experimented with. According to some leprologists, the toxoid acted as a stimulus in the production of diphtheria antitoxin which in turn was supposed to neutralize the leprosy toxin, since it was thought that there was a close biologic relationship between the two diseases. After experimental study of this new treatment, it was not found to be so beneficial as had been reported. In fact, at the National Leprosarium in Carville, they found it to be dangerous in the treatment of leprosy.

So, we've experimented down through the years and are now in the sulfone era. The papers are being conservative about the whole affair. We've all been fooled too many times. Here is their coverage of our new program:

+ New treatment for leprosy finds a skeptical reception.

+ With the announcement of the use of Promin as a treatment for leprosy, a faint hope has come to some of the world's 3,000,000 or more leprosy patients.

+ Experiments with this sulfa drug were made at the National Leprosarium at Carville, LA. Scientists there said that after three years of these tests, more than one half of the patients treated showed "definite improvement . . ."

+ First to work? If this new method proves itself safe and of real benefit, it will be the first such treatment to make good in the 6,000 years during which records have been kept concerning the disease.

+ But doctors are wisely skeptical. Said Doctor E. A. Fennel, an eminent leprologist and a member of the Board of Hospitals and Settlement in Oahu: "Chaulmoogra oil was played up the same way years ago, but it hasn't cured any patients. So far, decent care, clean living conditions, good food and vitamins constitute the only practical treatment known."

Dare we disagree with the eminent doctor? Well, we do and we shall see who is right. I keep my fingers crossed as I say this, but as I said before, we on the island are carrying the torch of hope. I hope I haven't bored you with this long epistle!

With Aloha,

Sr. Wilma

Parades celebrating the lives of Mother Marianne and Father Damien

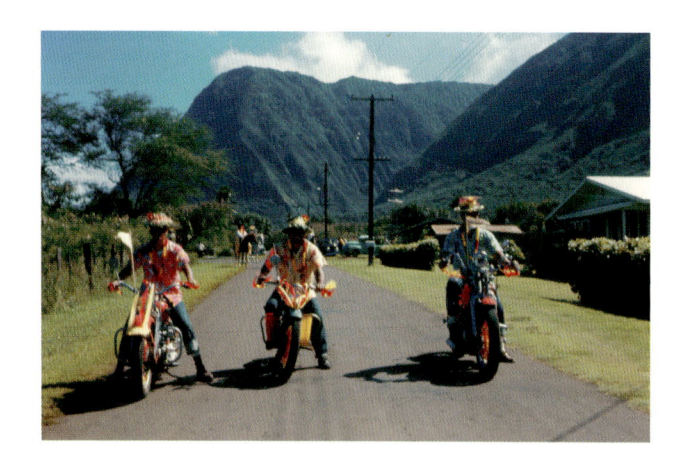

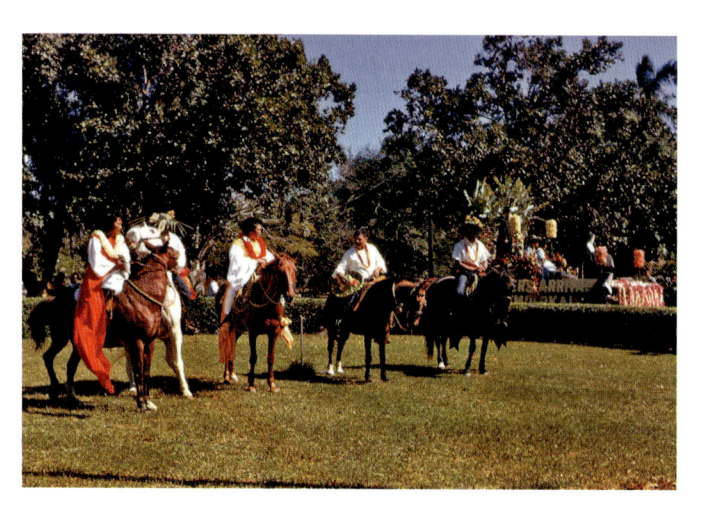

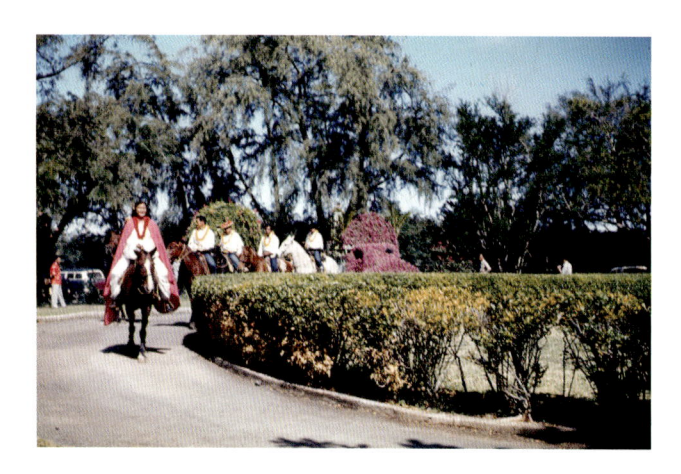

75

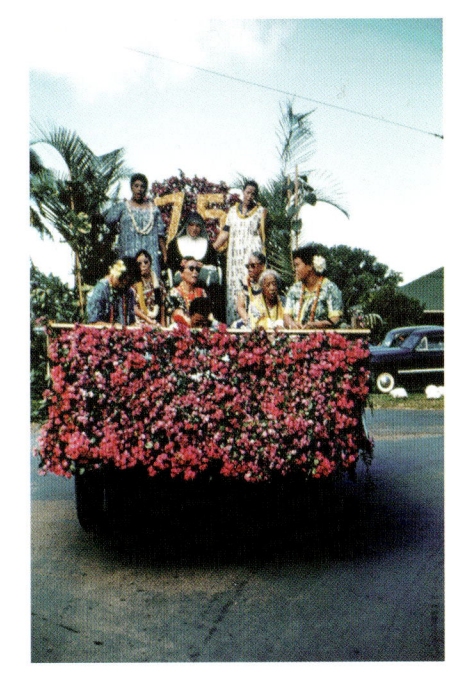

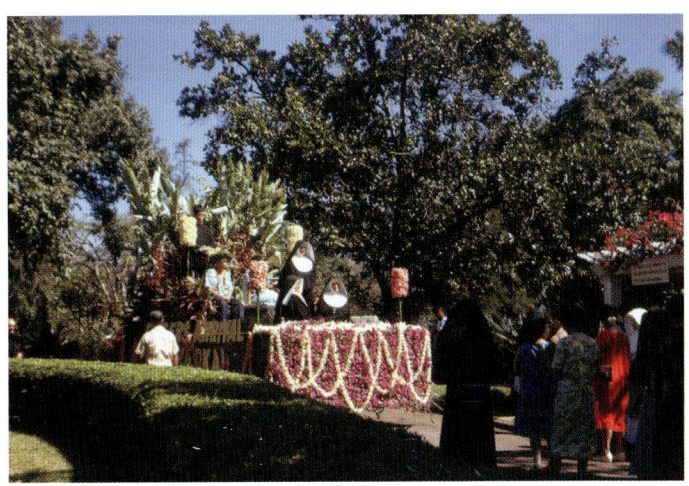

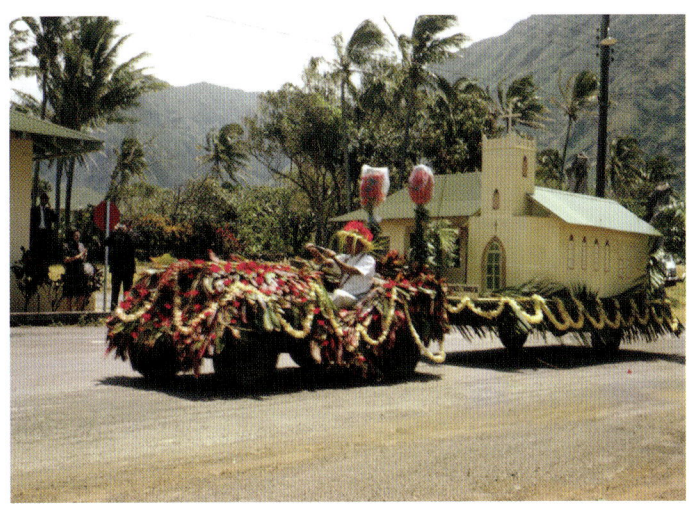

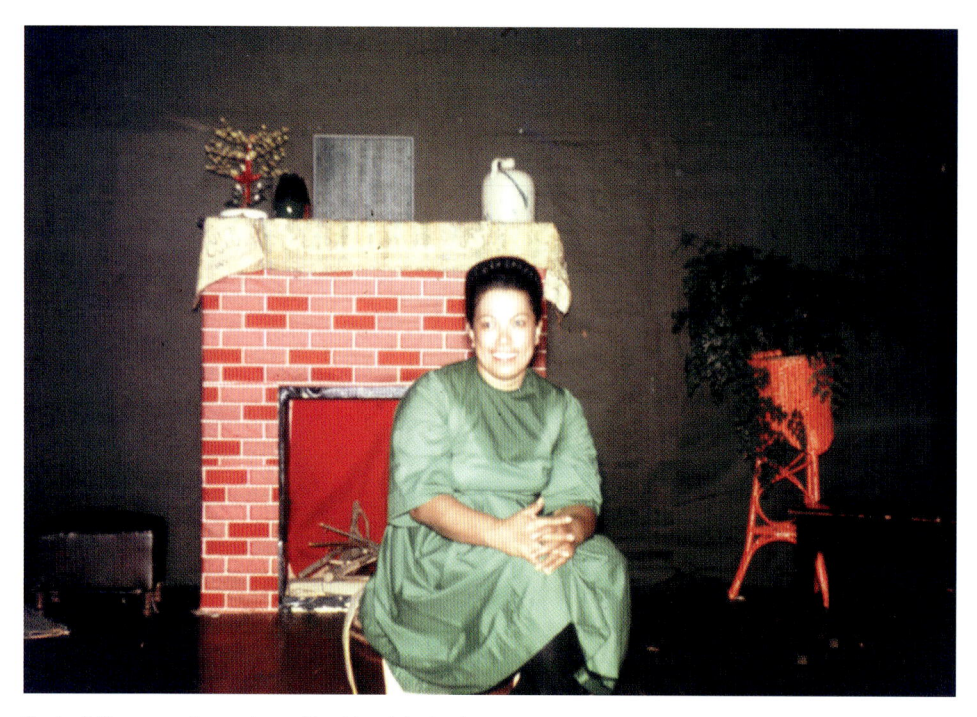

Kuulei Bell portrays the mother in "Amahl and the Night Visitors."

Dramatics: Kalaupapa Style

Dear Sister,

It's that time again: September. I have to decide what play we will present for Christmas this year. I'm quite sure that I'll decide on "Seven Nuns in Las Vegas."

I wonder whether the audience thinks about what goes on before a performance? I'll give you an example from our last production.

At Kalaupapa we have no proper stage now because it has been covered over by a huge cinema screen. So our dance floor is converted into a stage, and the small room adjoining the floor (which is used for storage) is cleaned out and converted into a dressing room.

I gave the order at dress rehearsal that everyone should be on deck an hour and a half before the performance. This was a mistake because, contrary to what I had expected, all arrived on time. So I suddenly found myself between two yelling, milling groups – one side the women, the other side the men. The women yelling for the men to get out while they were dressing, and the men yelling that they had as much right to dress as the women – and if the wahines didn't like it, they could dress with their eyes closed! I tried to yell louder than the crowd, but didn't make it. So I gave up. Finally, everyone was dressed. I looked around to make sure everyone was dressed properly and saw someone without makeup. "Kenneth, come over here and put on your makeup!"

"I'm not going on stage with makeup on. I'm a man." This is his first time on stage.

"Close your mouth and stand still. If I catch you wiping this off, you're going to get it!"

I threatened.

He shuffled off muttering dire threats like, "This is the last time!"

"Sister!" someone yelled from the crowd, "The electrician is looking for you. She's over here, Jim."

"Sister, we overloaded the line and blew a fuse."

"Oh, no!" We made a hurried consultation on how the load could be lessened and Jim ran off to see if he could find a fuse that wasn't locked up.

From another quarter, I heard, "Sister!"

"Over here, Myra."

The prima donna swept her way through the crowd. "Sister, I have decided that I am not going to kiss THAT MAN on stage!"

"What do you mean, you're not going to kiss him? He is supposed to be your brother!"

"I don't care if he's the King of England! I'm not going to kiss him."

I wrung my hands and shoved off to find THAT MAN. "Mark!"

"Over here, Sister."

"Mark, I'm making a small last minute change. Instead of kissing Myra at your entrance, you will just put your hand on her shoulder in greeting, OK?"

"How come?" asked Mark. I could see him wondering how this play ever got off the ground with such a kooky director.

Then as I pushed my way back through the crowd, a jokester, feeling hilarious over nothing apparent, said to me in pidgin English, "Juliet! Juliet! Where you, Juliet?"

"Look you eye, Romeo," I replied in pidgin. "Whatsa mattah, you no can see?" This stopped him for the time being.

"Sister!" Howard, carrying a large birdcage, elbowed his way through the crowd. "Sister, I think this chicken is upset from all the noise. It just laid an egg. What should I do?"

"Good Lord, I don't know anything about chickens, Howard. Take her outside where it's quiet and maybe she'll stop laying." Howard went off with the squawking chicken.

"Sister! Sister!"

"What is it, Tom?" I wiped my sopping brow.

"Sister! I'm not going on the stage NAKED!"

"What?" I asked startled.

"Look at my legs! They're naked!"

He was a Roman soldier and was wearing the standard dress. It apparently just dawned on him that his legs were showing. "Good heavens, Tom. You're covered to the knees!"

"I'm naked. I'm not going on stage like this!"

We were 60 miles away from the nearest leotard and 10 minutes from curtain time. I looked around desperately for an inspiration and saw a piece of white cloth lying on a chair. I tore it into strips and wound it around his legs fastening it with tape. I hoped that the audience would think he was a wounded soldier as he walked into the forum.

The first curtain signal was given and I roared, "Silence!" For once, my voice carried. There was a profound silence and they all looked as though they were headed for the guillotine.

"Take your places on stage and say a prayer. Good luck." And the play began.

Since I've been here, we've done several Nativity plays, Brother Orchid, Lilies of the Field, The Passion Play, Amahl and the Night Visitors, and Don Camillo's Flock. When I produced the first play, I was enthusiastically telling the medical director about all the talent and he made the scathing remark, "These people are stupid. If we haven't been able to do anything with them, who do you think you are?"

Ha! We showed him!

Keep well and God bless you,

With Aloha,

Sr. Wilma

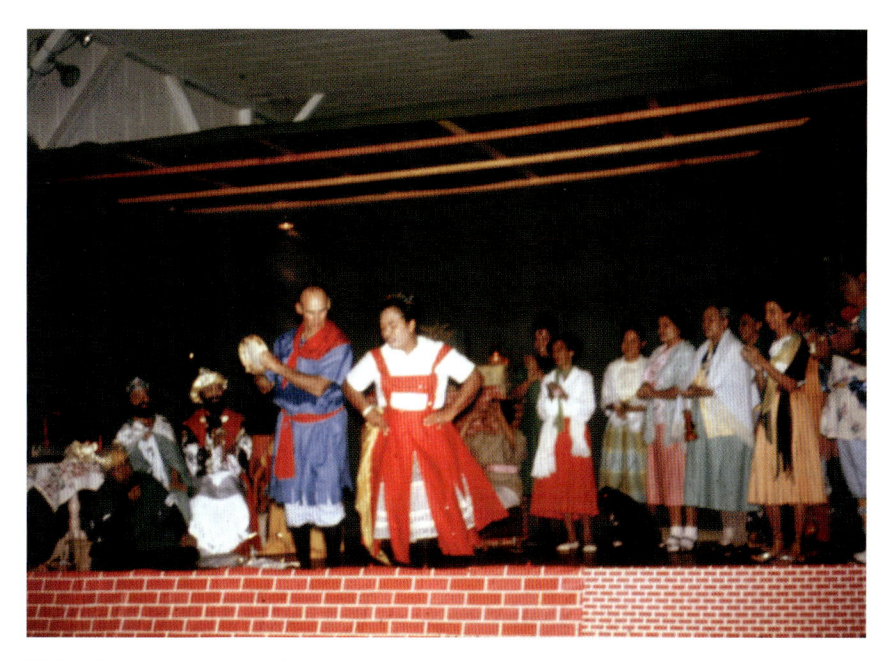

Night visitors being entertained.

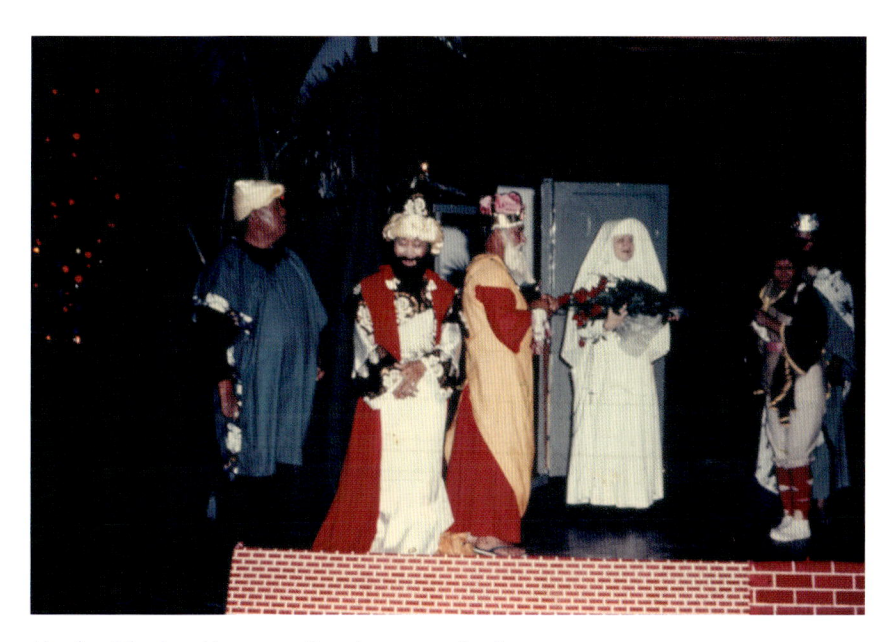

Ahmal and the three kings presenting a bouquet to the director.

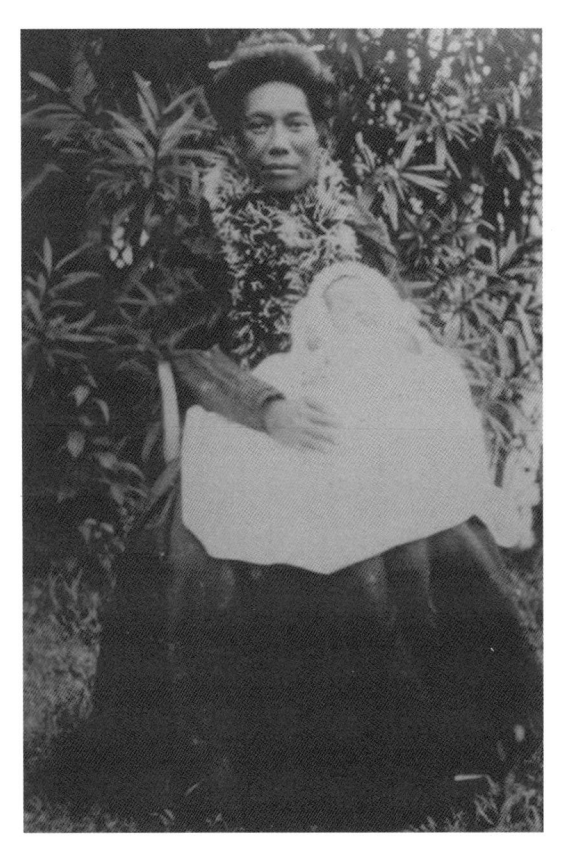

Mother and child, prior to separation.

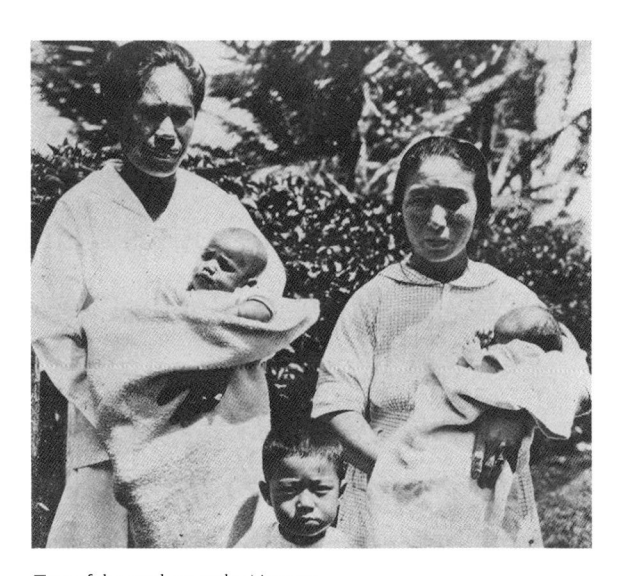

Two of the workers at the Nursery.

The Nursery

Dear Sister,

This is another beautiful day in Hawaii and my day off. I plan to practice on the organ in church for a few hours and pretend that I'm the Harp of God, playing beautiful music to the Lord. But I thought that I better answer your last letter before I start. I'm glad that you ask questions because there is so much to tell that I don't know where to begin.

You asked whether babies were born here. In the old days, yes. Now that transportation is more readily available, the mother is sent to Honolulu a few months ahead so that the child will not have a Kalaupapa birth certificate. It unfortunately brands the child in later life. The baby is taken from the mother immediately after delivery and from then on, she only sees the infant through a glass partition. It is felt that a baby is highly susceptible to the disease and no chances are taken on infection. I remember one of our prospective mothers saying to me one day, "I wish that I could carry my baby for more than nine months, Sister, because that is the only time that he will be mine." In the early days, the children were left in the Settlement with their parents, even if they did not have the disease. They were counted as patients on the census as the following letter describes:

                                                                      Kalawao, Aug. 15
                                                                       1877

Maj. Chas. Gulick
Secretary of the Board of Health
Honolulu

Sir:

. . . I beg you to do me the kindness to convey to his Excellency the President of the Board of Health the following facts, in regard to Kalua Wauahole

[w] so called, a minor living in the settlement and of whom information is required . . . .

I find that the child was born about the latter part of 1873—she Kalua [w] or [Kalua Waiahole] is now about 3 ½ years old. She was entered into the record of this settlement as a [patient] on Sept. 8, 1875 as the child of Awileko, a [patient] woman. Under the rules of the place, all the children born of [patient] parents are entitled to rations of food and are counted as [patients], and there are quite a few of these on our books who are receiving rations as if they were really [patients].

> I have the honor to remain
> Your obedient humble servant
> W. P. Ragsdale

In 1917 a nursery was built at the base of the pali in Kalaupapa, away from the densely populated part of the Settlement. The babies were taken here after birth, were kept for one year, then transferred to Honolulu, either to relatives or to one of the two homes built for these children by the government. The girls' home was staffed by our Sisters. At Kalaupapa, the nursery was staffed by two non-patient women who once lived with their patient husbands, now deceased. The parents were allowed to see their children on Sundays between one and four o'clock. Here also, the parents watched their children through a glass partition.

One of the old timers told me a story about the old nursery. Situated near the building was an ancient rock called "Pohakui" [swollen rock] believed to be a fertility rock. There were taboos connected with this rock. Any woman having her menses was forbidden to sit on the rock and defile it. If she did so, she would become bloated. Also, no dirty water was to touch the rock. Now, the workers in the nursery were in the habit of washing the diapers and throwing the water out and this flowed around the rock. The babies suddenly became ill for no apparent reason and some died. This was attributed to the defilement of the rock. When this water was thrown somewhere else, the sickness stopped. To the western mind this seems ridiculous, but according to the old timer, the fact remains that very odd things happened which could not be explained. Finally, a good Catholic volunteered to smash the rock, which he did. I was told that this stopped all the unusual happenings.

Since I am here we've had only one birth at the Settlement. An unmarried woman was admitted to the hospital complaining of abdominal pain. She would not let the doctor examine her so she was put to bed for observation. She was a very large woman and didn't show signs of pregnancy. That night one of the young nurses who came to Kalaupapa with me was on duty alone. About 7:00 p.m. the convent phone rang and I went to answer it. [Our phones are the old fashioned kind that you crank up.]

"Sister!" she shouted, "Marie just asked for the bedpan and when I picked it up, it had a baby in it! What should I do?"

"For heaven's sake, take it out of the pan!" I slammed down the phone and ran to the hospital. Needless to say, the baby aspirated fluid. Doctor and I worked on him with no luck. I took him to the convent and he died that night. I baptized him "Charles." I dressed him up and put him in a little coffin. He looked like a little angel. He is now in a far better place than he could ever have here. His mother did not fare so well. We found out that she had tried to abort him by crude methods and consequently she herself developed septicemia. She died a horrible death cursing God with her last breath. Lord, have mercy on her.

Well, Sister, I've given you a little idea of what goes on here. I'll give you more later. Now I have to retire to renew my bodily strength. Dawn seems to come earlier and earlier. So a fond farewell, and God bless you.

With Aloha,

Sr. Wilma

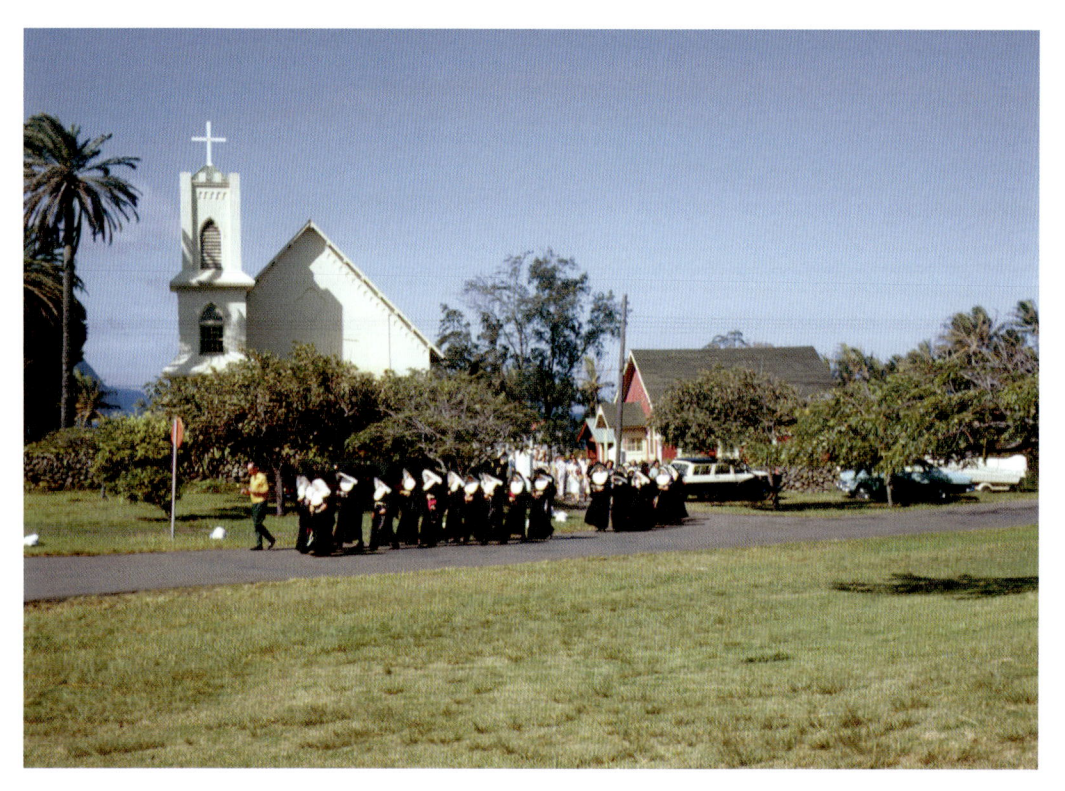

Beginning of Corpus Christi procession from Church to Bishop Home.

Religious Celebrations

1950

Dear Sister,

How time flies! We are already in the month of May – that wonderful month when all nature seems to burst forth with new life. How aptly it is called the Month of Mary who was the means of bringing to earth the new Adam, and with Him, the new life of the spirit. Tomorrow is Mother's Day, and all the Catholics are busy picking flowers to make leis for our Lady's statue. In the evening we will have a procession around the church with everyone carrying his or her lei to be presented. A sodalist will first crown the statue and then all the leis will be draped over it. The flowers will overflow to the altar. You should see the profusion of flowers: orchids, gardenias, ginger, plumeria, pikaki, and a host of others. To buy them would cost a fortune, and we just pick them out of our gardens!

After rosary and Benediction, we will have refreshments. There is a neat family spirit here.

Since we faithfully keep the first five Saturdays, as our Lady of Fatima recommended, the pastor thought that it would be nice to get a statue of our Lady of Fatima for the church, but he could never find one that he liked. So he told the Sisters to keep our eyes open and, if we found one, to let him know. I happened to go to Honolulu for vacation (we are not allowed to stay on the island for illness or vacation) and Sister Walter Damien said one day, "You've got to meet old Pete. He's the most eccentric old codger but fascinating. You'll love him!"

What does he do?" I asked.

"Oh, he's a little gaga on religion but harmless, and since his family has loads of money, they set up a religious store for him and he happily sells religious supplies."

I was surprised because I thought that we had only one religious store in Honolulu.

"What's the name of his store?"

"Oh, it's no store. He's got the stuff piled all over the house and in a Quonset hut on the property."

It sounded like a very interesting day. So we started out. The house looked as though it could collapse any minute and the grass was up to our knees. I began to have misgivings but we were admitted as long lost cousins. You have no idea of what the place looked like, Sister. Religious articles were piled under the bed, in the closets, in the dresser drawers, all over the floor. The amazing thing was that he knew where everything was. I asked if I could look around and he said, "Certainly."

So, while I poked around in unlikely places, he and Sister talked. I opened a door to a room which was pitch dark and brushed against a figure standing by the door. I let out a yell which brought the others running. Pete snapped on the light and I found myself looking into the face of the most beautiful Lady of Fatima. "Oh," I gasped, "I want to buy her, Pete."

"She's not for sale, Sister," he replied.

"Not for sale. Why?"

"Because she's my girl friend. I talk to her and she talks to me," he said in a manner which implied that the discussion was closed.

"Oh, but she belongs on Molokai. Think of the poor patients without our Lady of Fatima!"

"You can always buy another one," he answered sourly.

We argued for a long time and I finally broke him down, but I felt bad about it because he was so crushed to be losing his good friend. He put his foot down on one point. "She can't travel alone. I'll bring her to Molokai myself." I agreed and we sealed the bargain. Now the exquisite Lady stands on one of our altars watching over her children on Molokai.

We are now in the process of building a grotto to our Lady of Lourdes in what was formerly an unsightly gulch directly behind the rectory. The patients have dug up the ground and leveled it off to transform it into a beautiful park. I have drawn the plan for the grotto. I'm patterning it on the one we had at the Motherhouse when we were youngsters, remember?

The patients are doing all the work in their free time after working hours. They painfully haul huge rocks from the beach and acquire many bruises in the process. It is a labor of love and I'm sure that they will be rewarded by our Queen who is not outdone in generosity. When it is finished, I will send you a picture of it. I guarantee that it will be the loveliest grotto in the islands.

Last month we celebrated the anniversary of Father Damien's death. We had a High Mass at the church in Kalawao and after the services, there was a luau for the whole Settlement including invited guests from the other islands. A luau is a feast which you don't attend if you are counting calories. The main dish is the pig. The size depends on the crowd being fed. We usually have a 300 pound pig. The imu, a pit in which the food is cooked, is dug the night before. Then the animal is prepared. The pig is placed on ti leaves, under which is a burlap bag and chicken wire. Rocks are heated until they are red hot and then the cooks plunge their hands in ice water and quickly place the rocks in the pig's cavity. The other food which is to be cooked, such as yams, is placed around the pig. This is securely wrapped in ti leaves, then chicken wire and burlap. The food is then covered over with dirt and allowed to cook for about eight hours. When the finished product comes out, it is so tender that it falls off the bone and the taste is delicious! Along with this is served spinach cooked in coconut milk and squid, poi, lomi-lomi salmon, raw fish (red and white called sashimi), raw crab, and opihi (a clam which we pick off the rocks and is very expensive to buy). We are lucky; we just go to the seaside and pick them. The dessert is haupia, a special dish made from coconut. In the convent, I'm the only one who can eat all this without getting sick and I have a wonderful time!

Our next celebration will be Corpus Christi. The whole congregation will process from the church all the way to Bishop Home where we will have Benediction and then have a party. So life here is not all drudgery. I hope you can arrange your visit to coincide with one of our celebrations which are many. You'll love it. Well, Sister, until next time, may God gather you under the shadow of His Wings and keep you as the apple of His eyes.

With Aloha,

Sr. Wilma

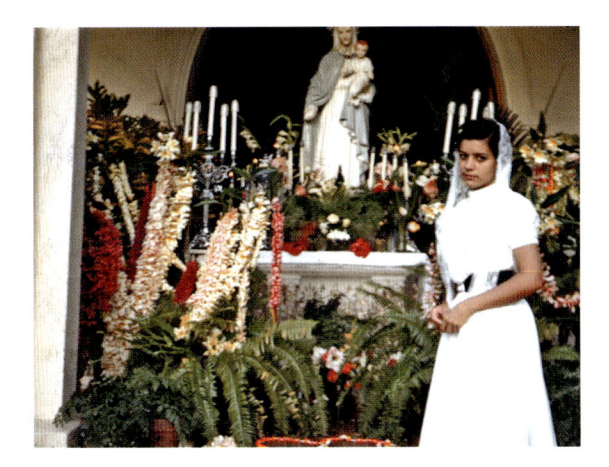

Mother's Day, Winifred Harada.

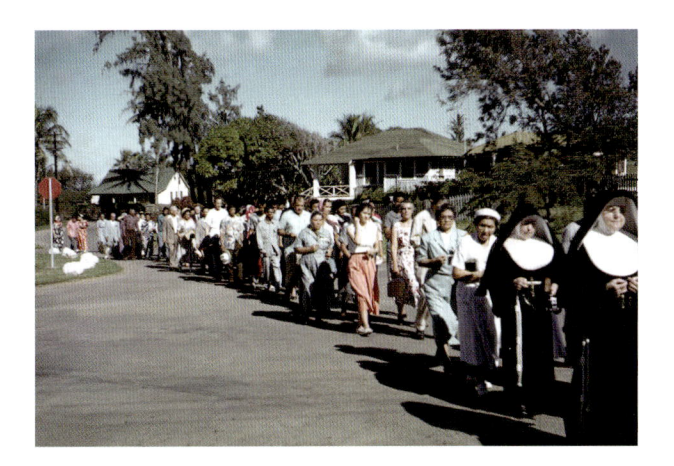

Corpus Christi procession.

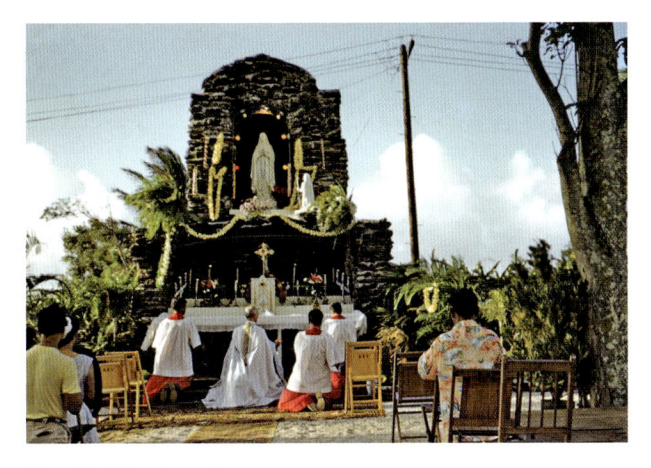

Grotto built by the patients.

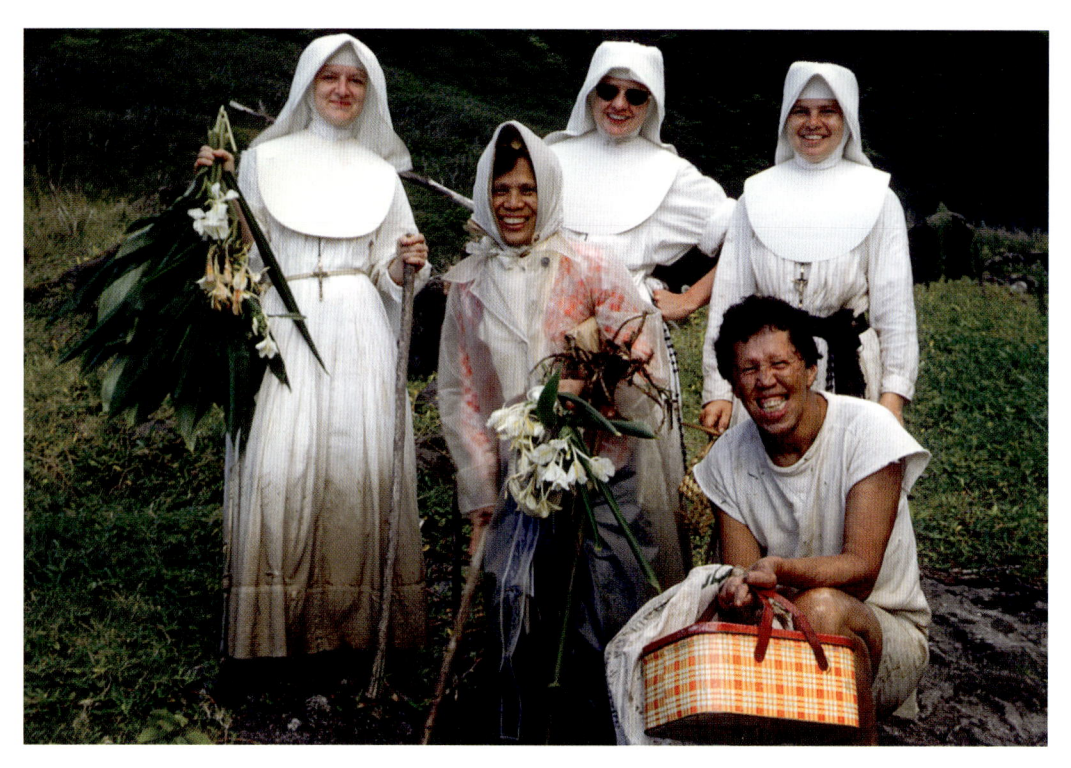

End of a perfect outing in Waikolu – tbe flowers are wild ginger.

Recreation

Dear Sister,

Another beautiful day in Hawaii. This was my day off so I spent it trudging the plains, checking out caves, and looking for artifacts. We have some very interesting caves that I know of. There is one in the mountainside that I haven't seen but would like to. It is a large burial cave apparently for the Alii. Another interesting one has a huge vaulted ceiling. It has three steps leading down to it and on the far side there is another hole. If one gets down on hands and knees, one can crawl through a tunnel and there is another cave with shelves on both sides. Perhaps sleeping quarters. We also have what the Hawaiians call "breathing caves" which means that periodically they open and close. There is one on the crater that has feather capes and helmets.

There is one that I would very much like to explore. One has to enter it in a boat when the tide is low. It is a long tunnel extending all the way to the "flats" I'm told. In it are canoes and other artifacts. Our "Old Ladies Cave" is the best known. At one time it extended from the crater to an opening high up in the cliffs overlooking the sea. The story is that one day war canoes coming from the island of Hawaii and on their way to Oahu, saw two old women sitting at the mouth of the cave. The warriors disembarked, poured water over the ground, and built a fire which caved in the earth. The warriors killed everyone in the tunnel. Nice people, aren't they? We still drop in from above. To prevent accidents, Sister Claudia and I marked the spot with a cow's skull.

Once, as we were walking along looking for something interesting, I saw an unusual bench carved out of stone.

"Oh, look at that beautiful love seat!" I said and went over to sit on it. It was the most comfortable chair that I ever sat on. I really fell in love with it. We took pictures of it. Then we walked on a few yards and I said, "Let's go back to look at that chair again." We turned around but there was no chair in sight. We searched but never found it. The picture we took of the chair came out beautifully, but the actual chair, we could not find again.

Of course this place is also a fisherman's paradise. If I am not exploring, I go fishing. A few weeks ago, I went out in a boat to troll. Suddenly I got a strike and began reeling the fish in. The boys began to laugh and I couldn't see what was so funny. All of a sudden the line went slack and I yelled, "Oh, I lost him!"

"Keep reeling the line in, Sister!"

"I told you, I lost him!"

"Reel the line in!" So I did and suddenly a bloody mass flew through the air and landed in the boat. I almost jumped out.

"What happened?" I asked as I stared at the large, bloody head of a fish.

"While you were reeling him in, a shark was chewing off the other end." I had visions of the shark taking a chunk out of the boat to get the rest of his meal.

"Let's get back to shore, pronto!" I said.

I took the head to the hospital and asked Mori the cook to make fish head soup for the patients. They love fish head soup. I weighed the head and it weighed eight pounds. A good size.

Another day, John decided to set a net for lobster. This is a true story but I'll embellish it a bit. It being a good day, John gathered up his gear and jogged happily to the sea, set his net, and went away.

By and by, along trundled a lobster. "Boy, oh boy, a free handout," said the lobster, and before he knew what happened, he was caught. Life became a nightmare of mazes. While he was frantically trying to repair his folly, a rakish rock bass cruised by.

"By Jove! What's that? A lobster?" He did an about turn and dived into the trap. We now have two greedy fish caught in an embarrassing situation. It being a halcyon day, a great many fish were out for a swim.

Soon a lovely large tuna hula-ed by. "Ciel! Est possible?" fluted the tuna. "Monsignor Bass for the taking?" With a few graceful swishes of her tail, she glided toward the net.

"Prenez garde!" yelled the rock bass, too late, as she crashed into the net.

"Ouf! Fi donc le coquin!" the tuna screeched as she thrashed about. The deep voice of the lobster was heard above the din, "Ferme! Mademoiselle, you're rocking the boat!"

Suddenly a shark zoomed by and then scrunched to a halt. "Zounds! It looks like a free meal back there!" and he crashed the net.

Meanwhile, back at the shack, John decided that it was time to check the net. Imagine his stupefaction when he came up with that catch of fish. John was very generous and shared some of the catch with the sisters and we had a delicious meal that night.

It just proves the old saying, "Everything comes to him who waits." Will write again soon. God bless you.

With Aloha,

Sr. Wilma

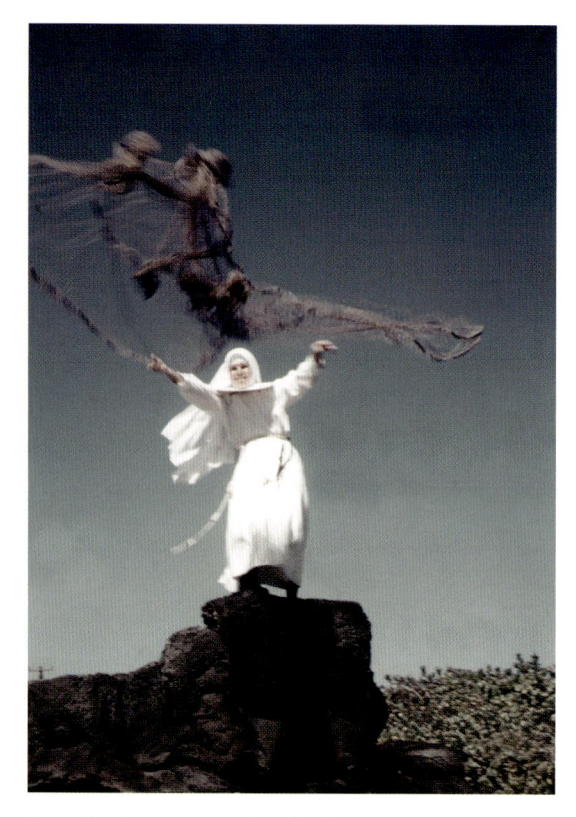

Sister Claudia not quite making the throw.

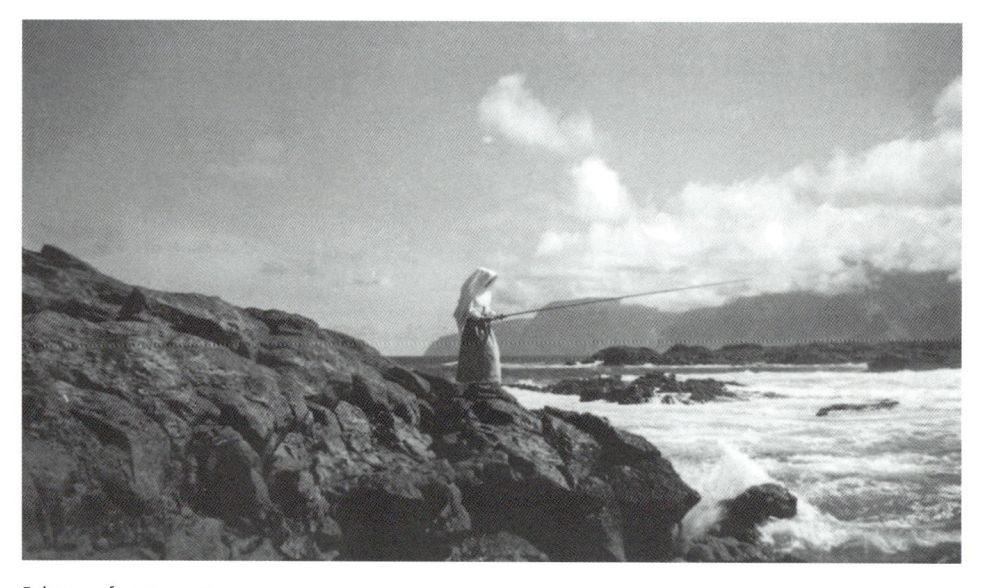

Fishing - a favorite pastime.

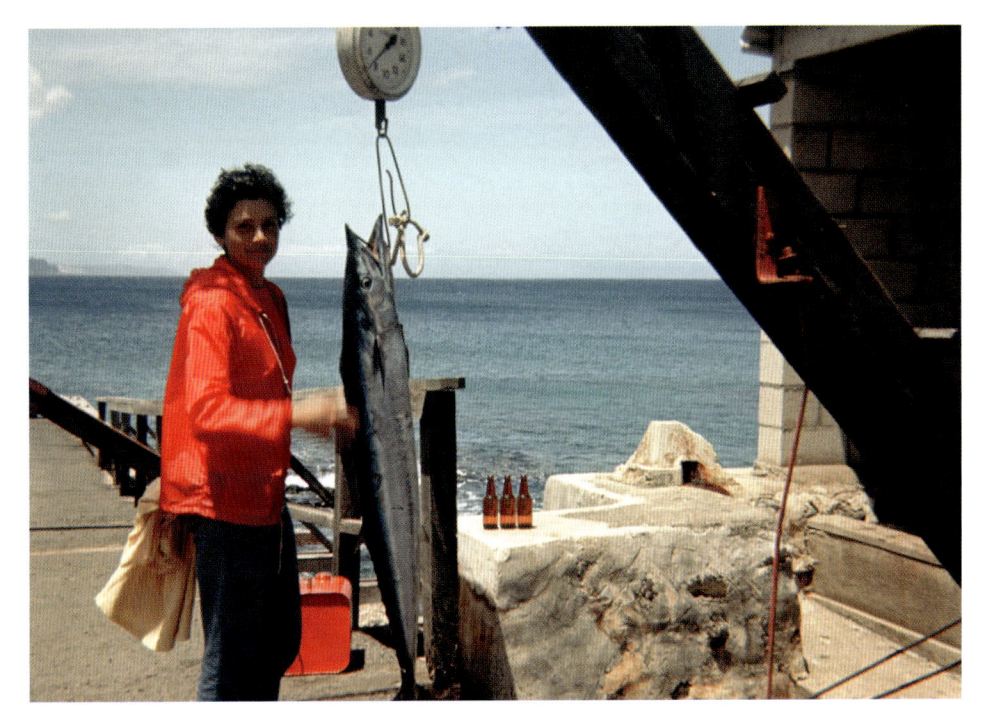

Winnie Harada displaying her catch of the day.

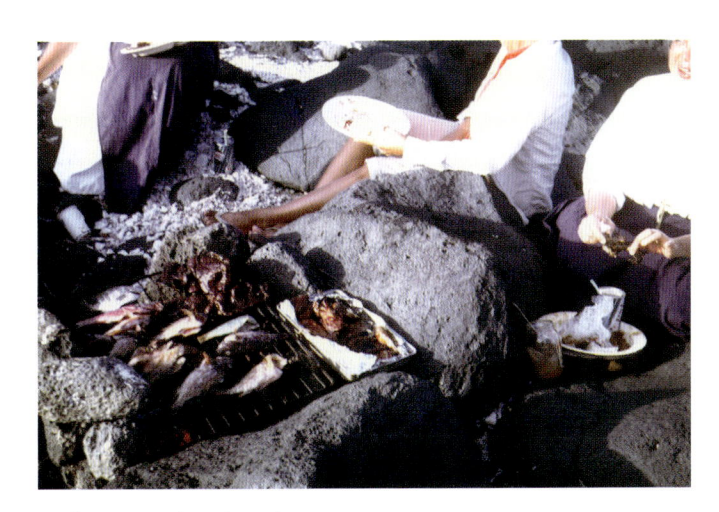

Cooking our catch on the rocks.

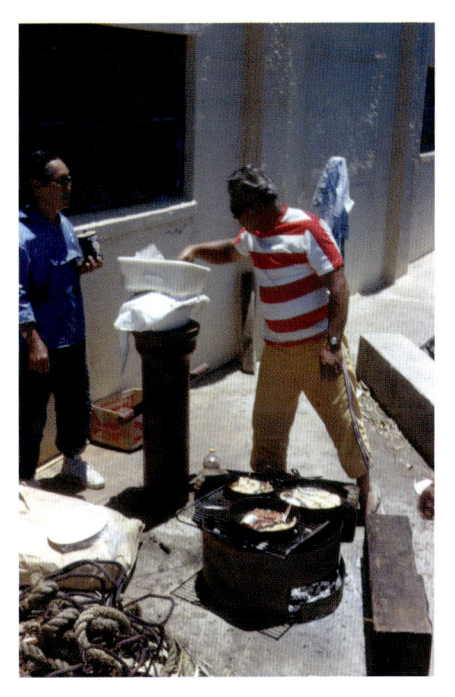

Chow time.

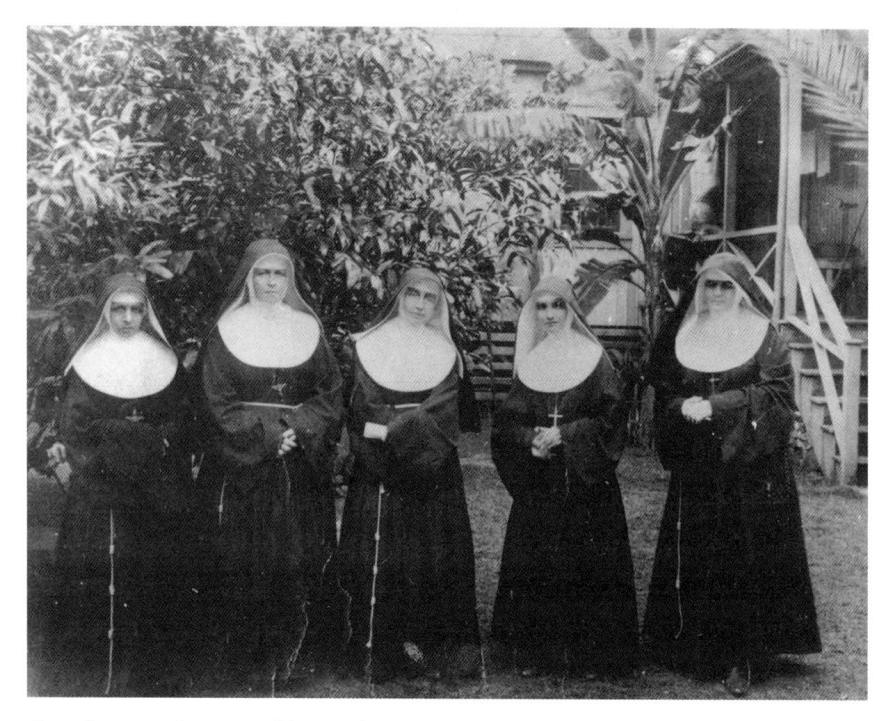

Sister Crescentia, Sister Leopoldina, Mother Marianne, Sister Elizabeth and Sister Vincent.

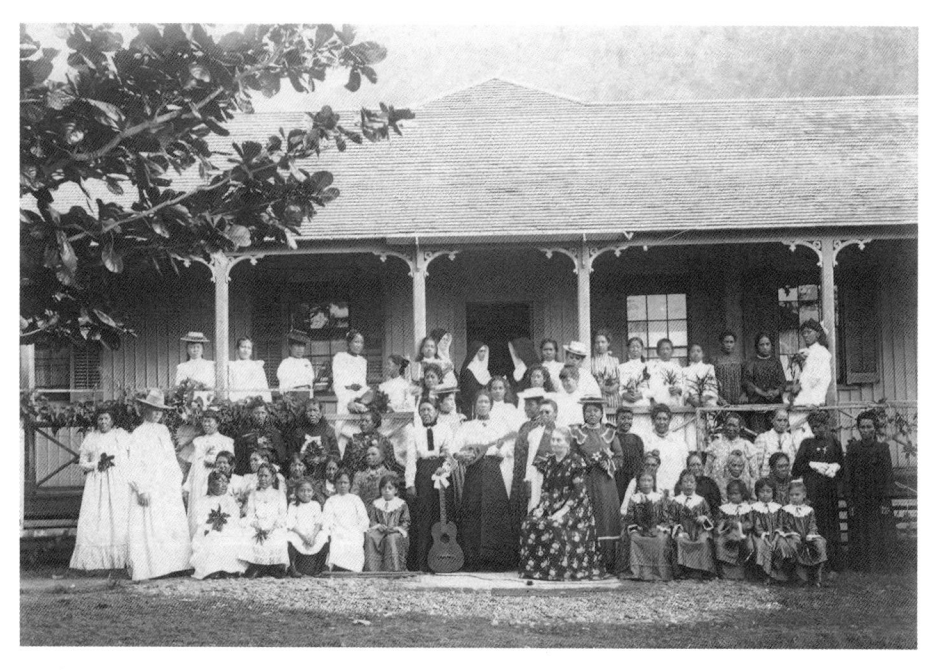

Bishop Home - c. 1904. With the women and girls are (left to right) Sister Leopoldina, Sister Elizabeth and Mother Marianne.

Early Beginnings

Dear Sister,

How did our Sisters happen to come to Molokai? Well, long ago on the distant island of Oahu, King David Kalakaua known as the "Merrie Monarch" sat at a table one fine day with his advisors and discussed a serious problem in the kingdom, the lack of nurses willing to work with leprosy. Following discussions between King Kalakaua and his Prime Minister, Walter Murray Gibson, it was decided that Father Leonor, noted for his diplomacy, would be sent to the States to recruit, if possible, Sisters for the task. He was at the point of giving up the mission as a failure when a little community of Franciscans in Syracuse offered to send Sisters, and so, Mother Marianne and six Sisters began the work of the community in the islands. They worked in the islands, first at the Kakaako Branch Hospital for Leprosy for five years before they were finally given permission to go to Molokai. The hospital at Kakaako was to be closed and a benefactor had been found to give funds for a women's home at Molokai. At last, Mother, who had planned to go to the Settlement from the beginning, had her wish fulfilled. This is how it came about:

April 18, 1888

Honorable C. R. Bishop
Honolulu

Sir:

I have the honor to acknowledge the receipt of your communication of the 13th inst. wherein you request the privilege of erecting buildings for women's and girls' home, at the . . . . settlement at Molokai.

In reply I beg to say that your generous proposal has been laid before the Cabinet and the Board of Health and is by them cordially approved.

I am also requested to extend to you the hearty thanks of the Cabinet and the Board of Health for this timely assistance, which will relieve one of the greatest necessities existing at the . . . . settlement.

                                      I have the honor to remain
                                      Your obedient servant
                                      L. A. Thurston
                                      Minister of the Interior

                                                  May 21st, 1888

Sister Marianne
Mother Superior Franciscan Sisters
Honolulu

Dear Madam:

The fact is no doubt well known to you, that one of the great hardships at the Molokai Settlement, has been the lack of a proper separate residence for the single women and girls. This difficulty seems now in a fair way to be remedied as far as the necessary buildings are concerned, through the generous offer of Honorable Charles R. Bishop, to provide a home for women and girls, including a suitable residence for those who may have charge of the same.

But such a home will not accomplish its end if it is not well ordered and governed. From the self-sacrificing example of yourself and the other Sisters of your order who are now ministering to the [patients], the Government has been led to hope that others of your order might be willing to assume the charge of such a home.

The duties to be discharged are of such a nature that I do not feel that I have the right to urge the matter upon you, or even to ask that any woman should devote herself to such a work. I will therefore confine myself to saying that the construction of such a home will be immediately proceeded with, to be ready for occupation in say three or four months from now.

The number of women and girls who will occupy the Home cannot be definitely estimated, but it will probably be in the vicinity of 100, with a possible increase to 150. The number of Sisters who would be needed in connection therewith is a matter which you are more competent to decide than I am, but it seems to me that six or eight would perhaps be a proper number.

If there are any members of your order, or of other orders having similar objects in view, who would be willing to undertake the charge of the proposed Home the Hawaiian Government will thankfully accept their assistance, and will do all in its power to aid and assist them, and in every way ameliorate the discomforts and difficulties of their position.

Any information which you may be pleased to give me concerning the likelihood of obtaining Sisters for this work will be deeply appreciated.

> By your humble, obedient servant,
> L. A. Thurston
> Minister of the Interior

So on November 14, 1888, at five in the morning, the Sisters and 42 seasick and tired patients leaned over the rails of the steamer Lehua to get a glimpse of their future home. At 8:00 that morning, Father Damien, who had been ill in bed for the past six weeks with a high fever, arrived at Kalaupapa to greet the Sisters. Their arrival seemed to revive him for awhile and he forgot his sufferings. Sister Vincent McCormick described their first visit to Kalawao made by her and Sister Leopoldina while Mother Marianne remained home to tend to the patients:

"We visited a house Father Damien began at Kalawao where there still were some small girls under the charge of a native Hawaiian. Father spoke to them in the Hawaiian language saying he was soon to die and the Sisters have come to take care of them, and that they must go to Kalaupapa, "by, and by."

"The children listened very attentively and when he had finshed his speech, two of the small girls ran toward him threw themselves on their knees and begged their good father not to send them away, but to let them stay until he would die and then they would go live with the sisters."

"The little girls kept their promise. As soon as the sick priest died and was buried, they came to us and died at Bishop Home."

"On a deathbed visit to Kalawao, Mother Marianne brought me with her as her companion, and I heard Father Damien's dying wish. Although he could not talk he managed to say in a whispering voice: 'Will you -- see -- to my boys when I am gone?' Three times he repeated the question. When he was promised affirmatively, 'the good Father was satisfied.' And this promise was kept."

This was the humble and fitting beginning for the work which the Sisters would undertake for many years to come. Life was primitive and harsh in those pioneer days. The Sisters' day began shortly after four in the morning. Sister Leopoldina did most of the soredressing while Mother Marianne concentrated on treating the patients medicinally, on the administration of the Home and the making of clothes for both the boys and girls at the settlement.

All was not misery and depression however. The Hawaiian people are a happy people. Twice a week the Sisters and the girls went for outings. On one day the group would hike into one of the beautiful cool valleys to pick mountain apples and other wild fruits. On another day they would go to the beach to pick opihi, a delicious Hawaiian clam. This reminds me of a story:

Mother Marianne and Sister Leopoldina spent many sleepless nights protecting the girls in the Home. Men were forever trying to break into the cottages. Mother always had a stout club ready behind the door of the convent so that at a moments notice, she could snatch it up and sally forth to do battle. Sister Leopoldina had a Bulls-eye lantern which she would keep hidden until she was ready to flash it on the one she wanted to see. This too reminds me of a story.

There lived in the Settlement a young man of high moral character. His sister, a beautiful girl, became a patient and came to Molokai to live with her brother. The men of the Settlement were constantly after her so that in desperation the young man asked Mother to admit Leilani to the Home. She was taken in immediately. However, this didn't deter the men. One day Leilani and a friend went to Mother Marianne. "Moddah, I get one plan for catch dem pilau kanakas. You help us, yeah?"

"What is your plan, Leilani?" asked Mother. Leilani outlined the plan and everything was agreed upon.

That night two men came to Leilani's window. "Eh, Leilani, you come out, yeah? We like see you."

"Eh, you guys like see me, you come in da hale [house]," answered Leilani. Her friend was standing by the door out of sight.

"Notting doin. Watsamatta, you loco or something? Da Wilikina [Sisters] catch us an we make die dead!"

"Da moddah awready moemoe. If you guys no like stay come in den pau stay, go you own hale." The men had no other choice and so they were lured onto the lanai. At this point, the friend ran to Mother who was hiding in the building.

"Moddah! Wikiwiki! We get em on da lanai!" Mother, clutching the club, and Sister Leopoldina holding the lantern on high, descended on the men with lightning speed.

"What are you doing here?" demanded Mother. The startled intruders turned to run. Mother, swinging the club, gave one a resounding whack on the back.

"Auwe!" he yelled.

"Give em a dirty lickin, Moddah!" the girls yelled gleefully. The other man, seeing the danger, ducked and as he came up, his head connected with the club knocking him silly for a moment. In the confusion, he lost his cap which was later used for evidence against him.

Mother's great care was the protection of the girls. This displeased some men at the Settlement so they made a plan to kill her. The women at the Home heard about their scheme and the night on which these men intended to come, they sat up all night armed with irons from their beds ready for battle. Mother Marianne herself retired for the night saying word must have gotten to the men that the women were not on their side and it was unlikely these fellows would show up. She expressed the hope no one would get hurt.

One would think that by this time the men would have given up trying to outwit the Sisters, but they didn't, so the Sisters had to be constantly on the alert to protect their girls.

Education was a "must" in the Home. The girls were given daily instructions by the Sisters. Besides formal instructions, they were taught embroidery and sewing. Dramatic and choral groups were also formed and the girls performed for visiting dignitaries. The young ladies also took their religion seriously because one day Father Wendelin came to Mother laughing. "Can you share the joke with me, Father?" asked Mother.

"Oh, Mother, I can hardly wait to spring a new problem on the eminent theologians. The girls just asked me if lice are meat or fish and if it was a sin to eat lice on Friday!"

The girls had long hair and an abundance of lice. The Sisters tried to keep this problem in check by making a mixture of brown soap and flowers of sulfur to wash the heads with. But the problem continued to be a constant one.

I would like to tell you a little bit about Mother Marianne. She was the vitalizing force in Bishop Home. All looked to her for support and comfort. She was very kind, but she was also very determined for all that concerned the welfare of the community and for all under her maternal care. Though she was a pillar of strength to others, she herself had no one to confide her heartaches to. She took comfort in prayer. She had a great faith in Our Lady of Lourdes and many still say that wonderful things were accomplished with the Lourdes water which she used for desperate cases in the Home.

As one reads her diary, one can glimpse what she must have suffered, being a refined, sensitive soul. The virtues which stand out in her life are her patience and charity toward her fellow beings. Through her kindness and charity, she gradually won over the unruly patients in the Settlement, and this made things easier for the Sisters. She practiced her charity quietly and was often severely criticized for her kindness to others. Once, after Mother had been publicly insulted, a Sister said to her, "Mother, how can you be so kind to him?"

Mother replied, "You can win them over more with kindness than with insult."

Mother was always a perfect lady. She was naturally soft-spoken and quiet and could not bear being in the company of boisterous people. She was ill most of the 30 years she spent on Molokai. She suffered intensely from migraine headaches, especially during the Kona weather. She was also subject to severe hemorrhages, apparently of gastric origin, but this did not deter her from being on duty ill as she was. When she was urged by the Sisters to rest, she would reply, "I must be a good example to others."

On August 9, 1918, at 4:30 in the morning, Mother was anointed and she died that night. They wished to bury her next to Father Damien's monument at Kalaupapa, but when they began to dig, they encountered solid rock so they buried her closer to the convent. Later, the patients erected a beautiful monument over her grave. Thus passed a great and noble soul from the shores of Molokai but her spirit remains and it is this spirit which continues to motivate the Sisters who try to walk in her footsteps today.

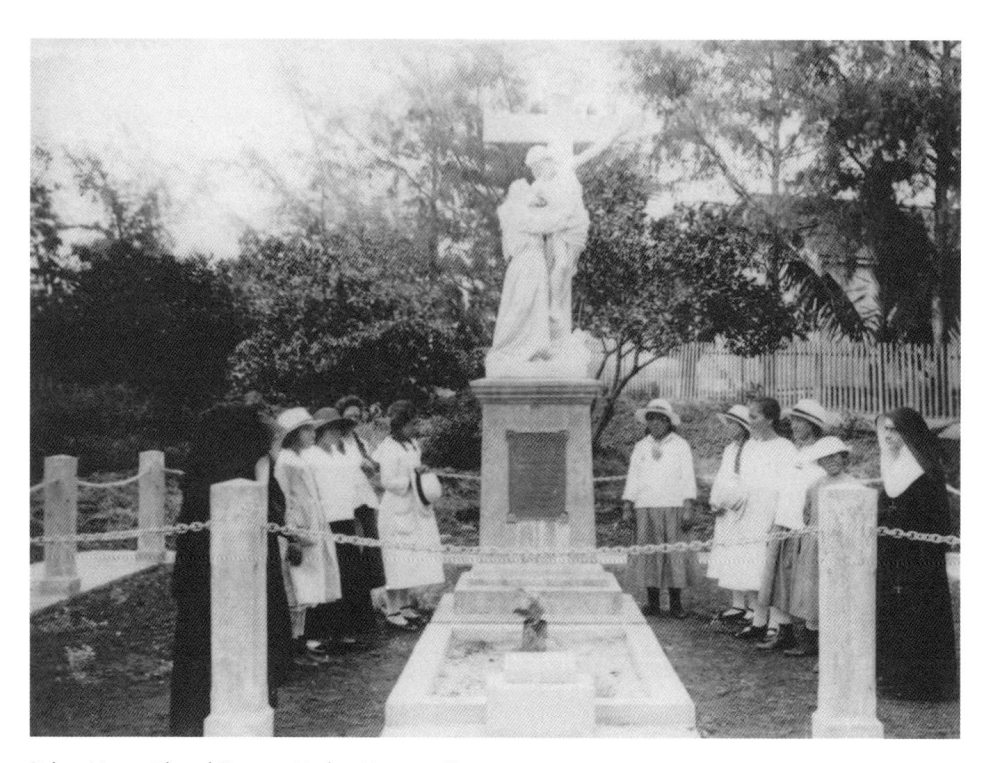

Bishop Home girls and Sisters at Mother Marianne Grave.

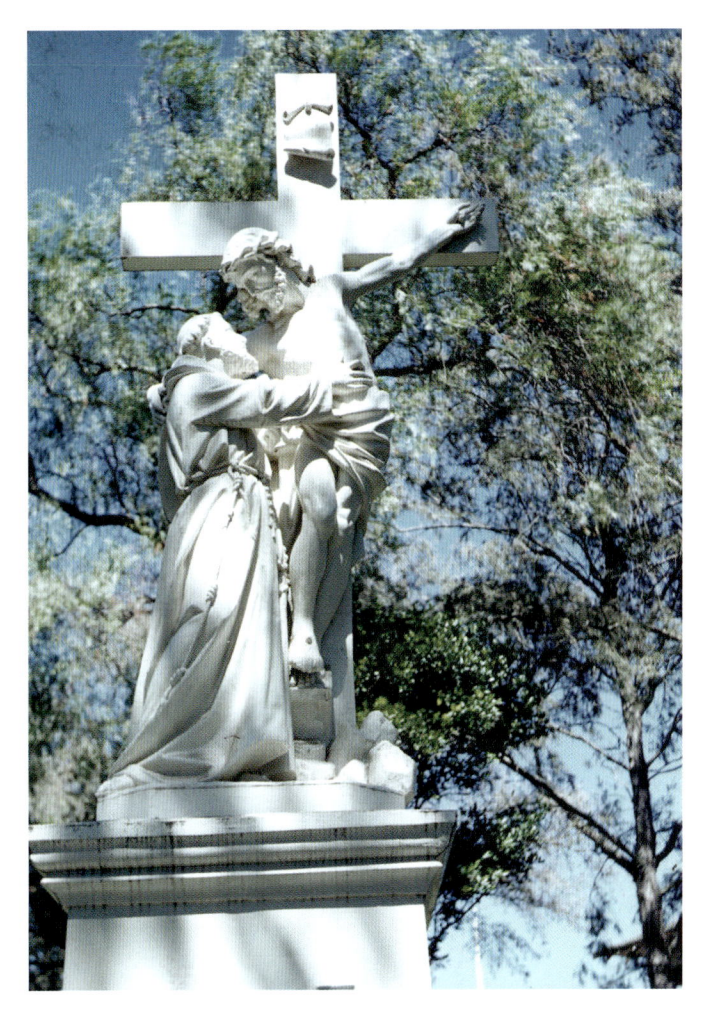

Monument over Mother Marianne's grave.

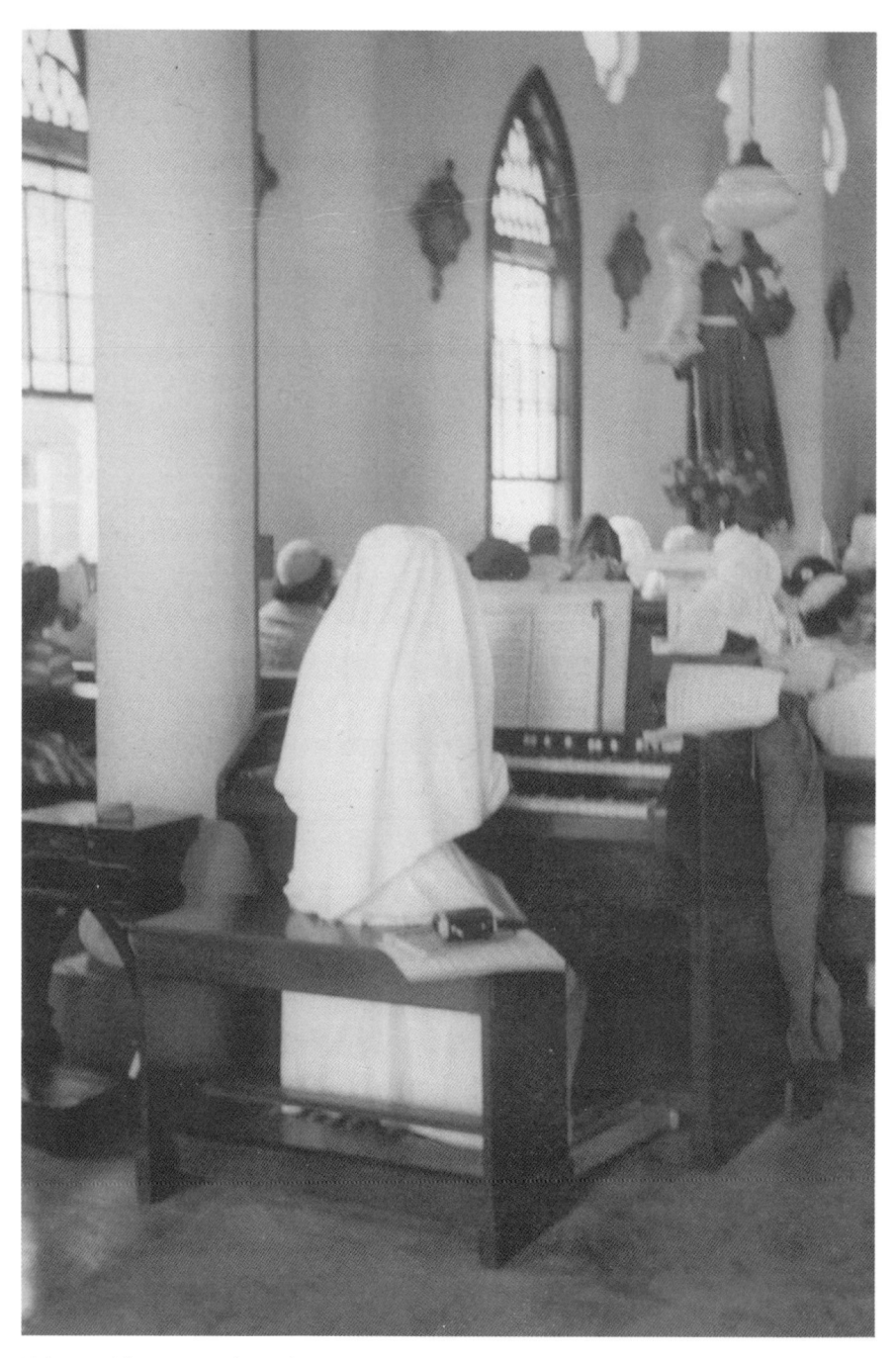

Making joyful music unto the Lord.

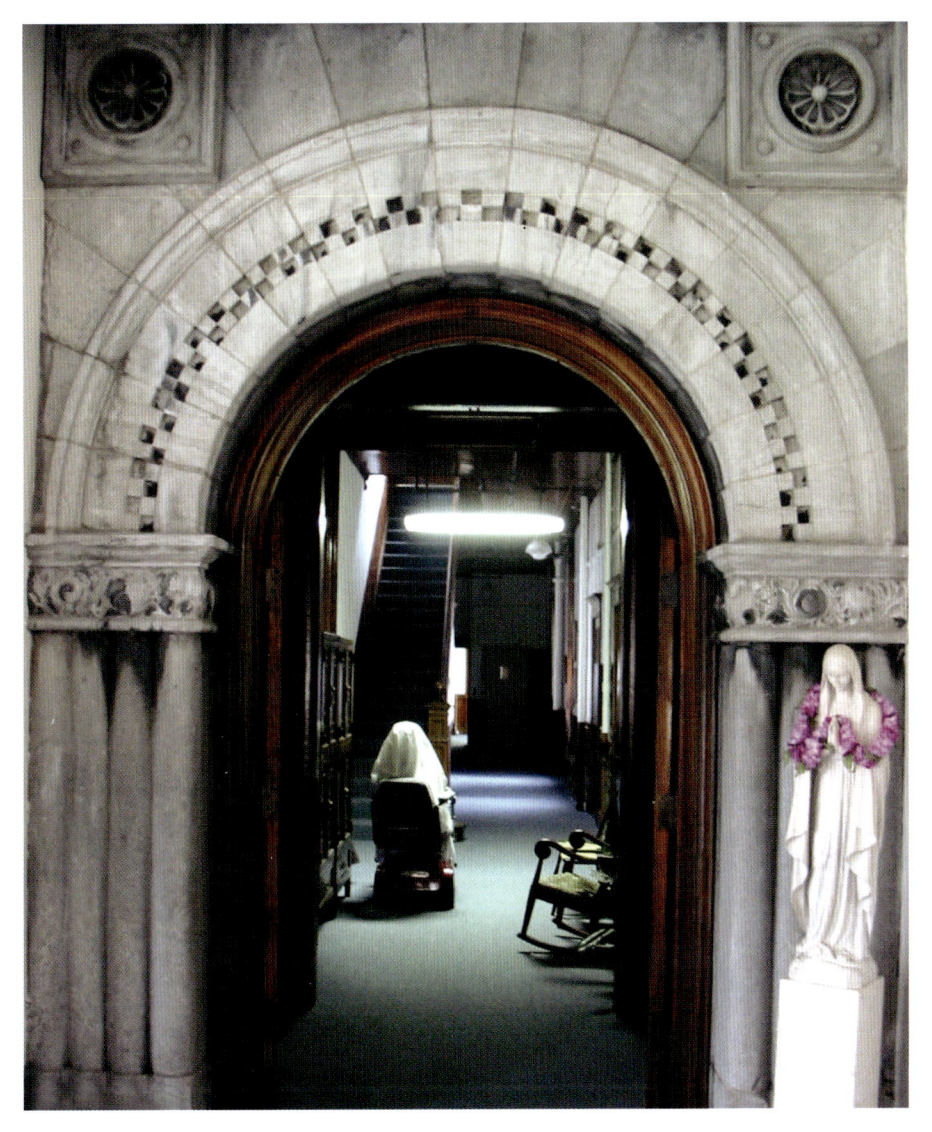

Sister Wilma at the Mother House of the Sisters of Saint Francis in Syracuse, New York. *Photo by Henry Law*

"The shades of evening are gently descending on another day as I write this, and we are one day closer to eternity. Time seems to fly on the wings of the wind on Molokai."

MOLOKAI

Oh far and lonely strand
Whose voice, once heard smoulders in the heart
And cries again for utterance,
I speak.
That out of many mouths
The world may know this place
Whose only wealth, disease,
Mounts with leaden swiftness unto death.
Here men seek solace in Omar's creed:
"O make the most of what ye yet may spend"
Or find answer in faith to a deeper need:
"Lift up your hearts, I am the End."

Molokai, against your bleak shore
Strewn with bitter sand
I will roll laughter,
Broad as your sorrow
Deep as your pain.
And down deep rutted lanes
Spill bright peace –
Bright as the breaking light
In eyes still wet
With childhood's sudden rains.

I will pile phrase on climbing phrase
To rear this barrier cliff
Then down its face
Eroded with the years
Pour brief cataracts of human tears.
I will cut chasms cruel
Deep in the tortured stuff of mortal hearts

And for a tool -- ?
Only the remembered touch
Of baby finger tips
On mother-lips.

I will fling noosed words
About all nothingness
Then drop the whole
Into your heart;

And as returning echoes roll,
Know I sought in vain
To fill a void
Greater by the measure of your pain.

But oh what traitor deed!
Words are not servant to my need.
This is a song of morning
And it still is night.
I have but shot the bird –
I have not captured flight.

But dawning –
He, Who with equal ease
Poised these mountains
Cupped these seas;
And with diviner art
Polished the facets
Of the human heart,
In words God-minted shall unfold
Your story, Molokai –
Till then – untold.

-- Sister Walter Damien

NOTES

Not all of this listing of references used by Sister Wilma can be found but most were located.

Books:

Page 69. Mouritz, Arthur. <u>The Path of the Destroyer: A History of Leprosy in the Hawaiian Islands and Thirty Years' Research into the Means by Which It Has Been Spread</u>. Honolulu: Honolulu Star-Bulletin Press, 1916.

Newspaper Articles:

Page 12 – 13. Dr. Bechtinger. "The Leprosy Hospital on Molokai." *P. C. Advertiser, 1867.*

Page 22. "Sampan Hits Molokai Reef in Whirlwind." Unidentified newspaper article, 1940.

Page 69 – 70. Untitled article. *Hawaiian Star.* April 13, 1903.

Page 73. Headlines from various newspapers in Hawaii. Circa 1946.

Hawaiian Mission Correspondence and Writings Collected and Preserved by the Third Order of the Sisters of St. Francis of the Neumann Communities:

Page 3. "A Song of Farewell." by two unidentified Kalaupapa residents, 1922.

Page 9. Untitled Letter. The Independent. Hawaii, 1869.

Pages 10 – 11. Letter to E.O. Hall from S.N. Holokahiki, December 25, 1873. Hawaii State Archives.

Page 17. Quote from Letter from Charles Bishop to R.W. Meyer, 1887.

Pages 17-18. Charles Warren Stoddard, <u>The Lepers of Molokai</u>. Notre Dame, Indiana: 1885.

Page 57. Dr. Nathaniel B. Emerson. "Da Very First Christmas." Christmas story as recalled by native Hawaiians.

Page 63 – 66. Medical Director's Speech. July, 1946.

Page 67. Letter from Resident Physician to Supt. Bd of Hospitals and Settlement.

Page 68. Letter from parents of resident to medical staff and employees of Kalaupapa Pali Station.

Page 70 – 71. Report by D. Dayton. "The Inspection of [Patients]." May 11, 1893.

Page 71 – 71. Information from unidentified sources about treatment of leprosy beginning with the Goto treatment.

Page 83 – 84. Letter to Maj. Chas. Gulick from W.P. Ragsdale, Kalawao, August 15, 1877. Hawaii

State Archives.

Page 99 – 100. Letter to Hon. C. R. Bishop from L.A. Thurston, Minister of the Interior, April 18, 1888.

Hawaii State Archives.

Page 100 – 101. Letter to Sr. Marianne, Mother Superior, from L. A. Thurston, May 21, 1888. Mother Marianne Cope Archives, Syracuse, N.Y.

Page 102. <u>Sister Vincent McCormick Journal</u>, Mother Marianne Cope Archives, Syracuse, N.Y.

Page 103. Remembrances from <u>Sister Leopoldina Burns Journals</u>. Mother Marianne Archives, Syracuse, N.Y.

Page 110 – 111. Wright, O.S.F., Sister Walter Damien, "Molokai."

Photographs Collected and Preserved by the Third Order of the Sisters of St. Francis of the Neumann Communities and A Colorful Contribution of Photos for Usage by Henry and Anwei Law.